THROUGH THE EYES OF INSANITY

SPELLBOUND INTO THE
CONSCIOUSNESS OF CHAOS

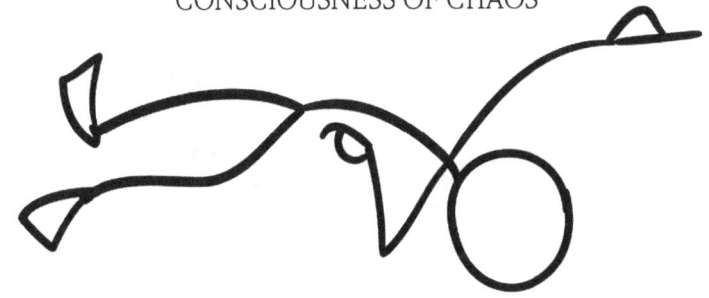

LORI S MOORE

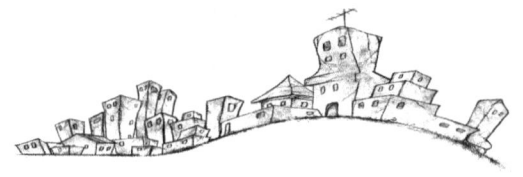

TO MY FAMILY
AND FRIENDS FOR
LOVING, THE
UNLOVABLE

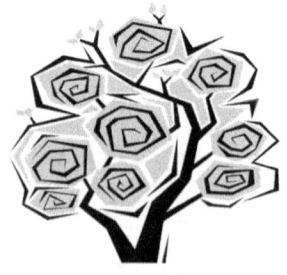

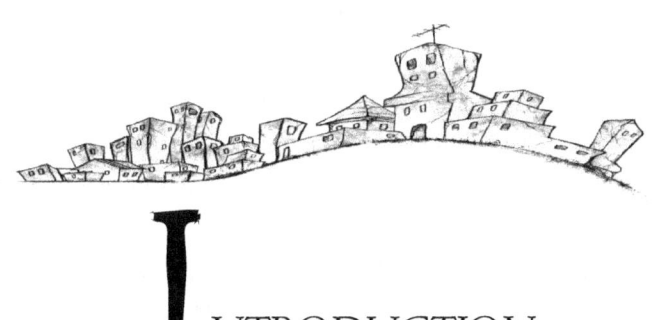

Introduction

Through the Eyes of Insanity draws you into a world seen through the eyes of mental illness. Its creation was based on actual memories, thoughts, and ideas that were transpired into a story that incorporates the power of emotion through poetry. It takes you on a journey within the broken mind by involving you with the struggles of mental illness in everyday life.

I have been diagnosed with ADHD, General Anxiety, Social Anxiety and Bipolar Disorder. This is who I am. I have many labels, but they do not define who I am as a person. They just represent the emotions I feel.

My hopes are to eliminate the stigma placed on mental health and to raise awareness of its impact. This memoir is about understanding the complexities, whether it is you or someone you know.

Mental illness has many faces that are often hidden. No one should have to hide who they are or feel alone.

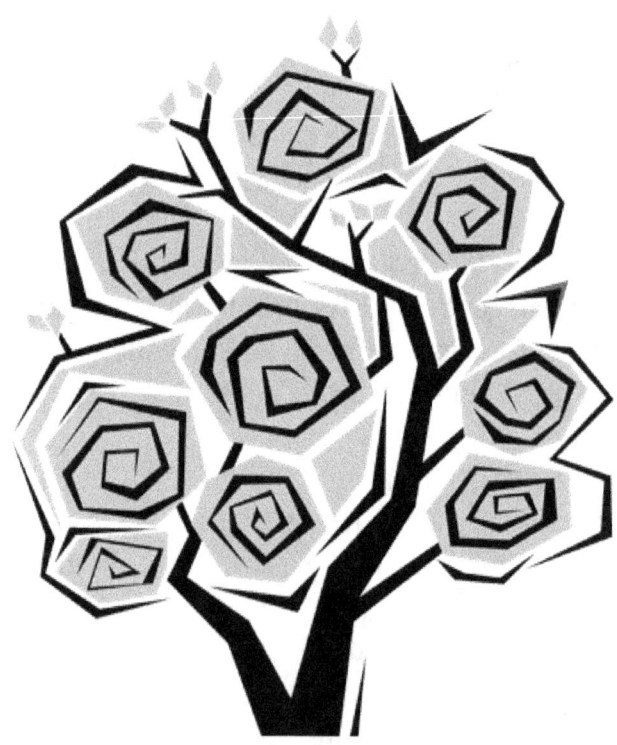

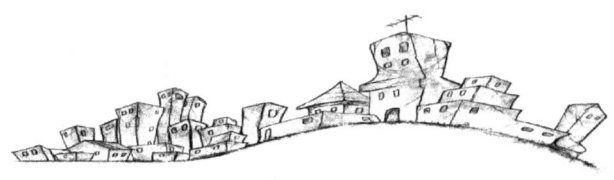

CONTENTS

SOMEWHERE IN THE MIDDLE 1

WHERE THE SHEEP ROAM 5

THE PORTAL 17

DARKNESS FALLS 28

THE ESCAPE 44

REJECTED 54

THE BLUE RUBBER RING 60

WALKING THE ROPE 73

CHOICES 81

LABELED 87

PINK ELEPHANTS ON PARADE 91

INTO THE VOID 97

THE WAR 108

THE WALL 118

RUN AWAY 131

WHERE ARE WE NOW? 139

THE IN-BETWEEN 142

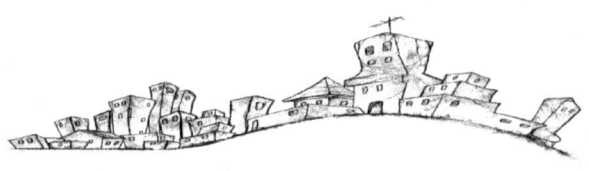

I *SEE DEAD PEOPLE*... 150

T*HE WORLD TODAY* 156

I*SOLATED*... 164

R*EALITY OR ILLUSION?* 170

W*HERE DO I GO FROM HERE?* 178

T*HIS IS NOT THE END*....................................... 185

B*ACK TO THE BEGINNING*............................... 191

W*HAT IS NEGATIVE CAN BE POSITIVE*........... 195

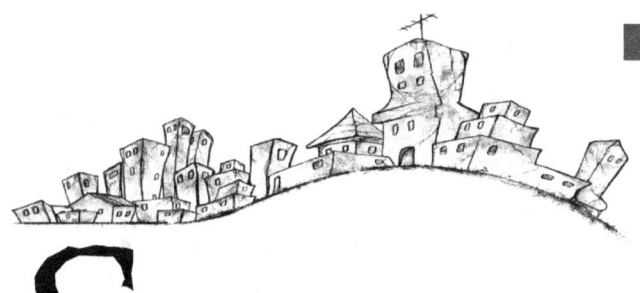

SOMEWHERE IN THE MIDDLE

You think you know me.
But you do not know me.

You do not know the extent
of the torment I feel,
Because I hide it every day.

I may look normal to you,
But I am broken inside.
I am lost within these walls.
A war I cannot win.

I cannot stand still,
I cannot stop the voices within my head.

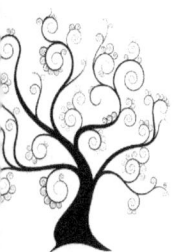

I am afraid to look around.
I am scared to talk.
I am afraid to walk.

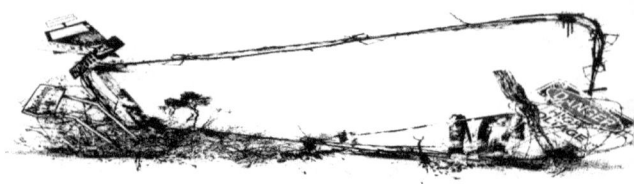

I am afraid everything I do is wrong.
My mind does not stop.
I see things that are not there.

I keep telling myself these things are not real,
But my mind is overpowering
lacking the sanity taken for granted.

I think people are always watching everything I do.
I am afraid.

I envision a knife piercing through every part of my body,
Slowly.

You think I am okay when you see me,
But if you looked deep into my eyes,
You would see the constant pain that I try to keep hidden.

I need everything in a specific place
And in a certain way,
To the point of obsession.

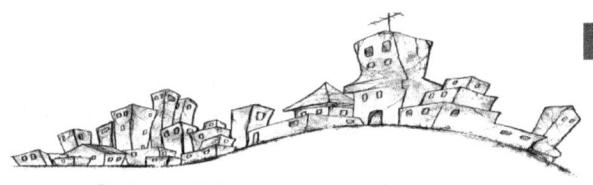

Only to fidget more and more
And become so uncomfortable,
It eats me from the inside out.

I tell myself to be resilient,
To cope,
To fight it.

I tell myself this to hold onto a glimpse of sanity,
Because it does not go away.

I do not understand why I am so broken.
The pain it hurts so much.

I try not to feel too much emotion because
when I do,
I become vulnerable and more susceptible to
what I cannot control.

My family and friends are my anchors.
They are what keeps me alive each day.
Each breath I take.
I take for them,

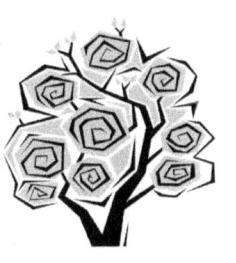

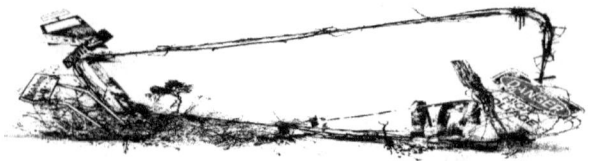

Because each breath I take gets harder and harder,
In every way.

The next time you look at someone and judge them,
Do not think they do not,
Struggle through each day.

Because you thought you knew me.
But you knew nothing,

Of the struggles that keep me alive.
To breathe another day."

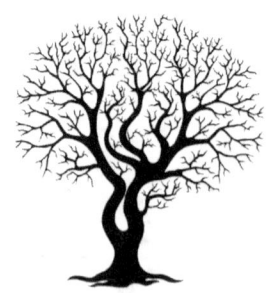

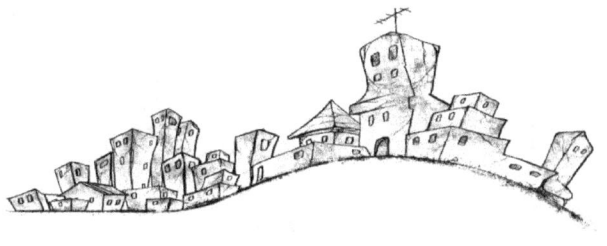

WHERE THE SHEEP ROAM

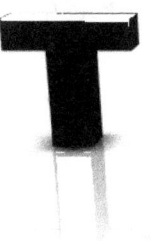

he sleeper sleeps until the hands move back.
Travelling through a vortex of black.

The walls explode with the memories that past.

Scattered and shattered the fragments remain,
Until you close your eyes and find you are not that sane.

I do not want to run.
I will not hide.

See the world with these contaminated eyes.

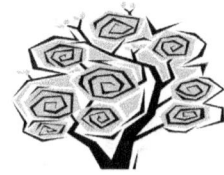

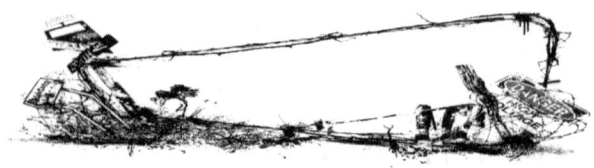

Bloodstained tears,
Coated with fears.

Watch the worlds indefinitely collide.
Underneath the emptiness of the cold moon shadow,
The burning star rises from far to the east.

Let light into your world,
Until the storms rage on.

Sending flashes of pain with a thunderous sound,
The sleeper sleeps in present time.

Forgetting the reasons why everything was left behind.
Buried deep protected and lost inside.

Only to walk towards a new dimensional line.
Unexpectedly, a thought comes back from a smell.

One by one, it gave me a reason to tell.

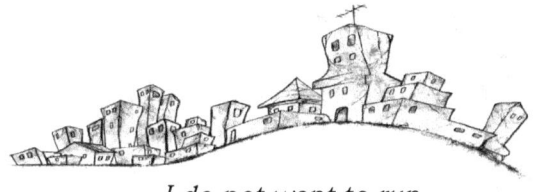

*I do not want to run.
I will not hide.*

*Watch my life through the vortex as the sleeper sleeps.
To awaken to find the fragments put back together,
Piece by piece."*

I will not conform to the human zoo, nor will I fit into its little box. My perception of the world is a mindset built mostly on observation that primarily decodes human behaviour. The fortified walls that I have built protect me from the harm of thy enemy.

Trust no one!

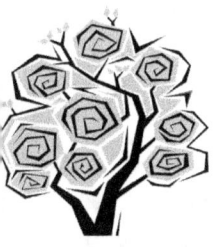

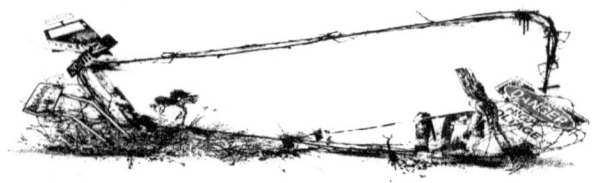

*"Judged are the superficial idiosyncrasies.
Spoken in riddles and jokes out loud.*

Hidden behind a lifetime of walls.

*Listen to the words,
No confidence,
No true strength.*

*Pushed the person that could have been,
Somewhere lost,
Somewhere deep.*

*Envision the words I enunciate.
Read between the scars.*

*Judge me not for my imperfections.
But who I scream to be out loud.*

*Torn from the inside,
Decipher my language,
Help show me who I am.*

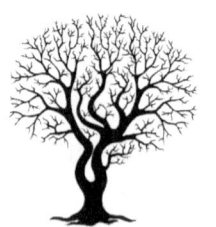

Tear down these walls.

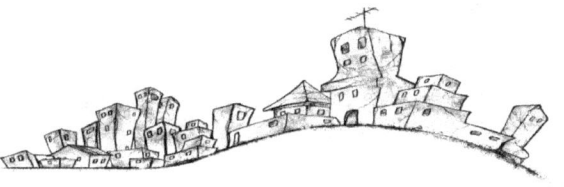

I do not want to fall.
Fall back down again.

Exude my confidence,
Make me feel alive.

Pull me from my fears.

I am lost,
I am judged.
Please take my hand.

I do not want to hide.
Listen to my words,

I am falling,
I am falling.

I need to get up.
Back up from the ground.
Help me!

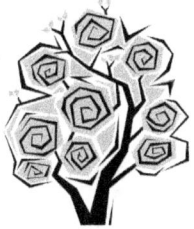

Help me get back up again.
So, I can meet the person,
I truly am."

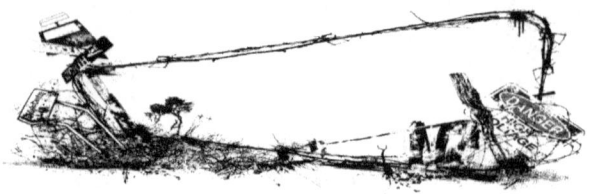

I will choke and vomit the foreign drugs shoved down my throat while locked in the padded cell. I will not assimilate and be a sheep that saunters aimlessly looking for my master to lead.

"They are here!"

"Why are you procrastinating?"

"You are delusional if you think these pathetic words will be read by anyone, no one cares!"

"Stop listening to all their negativity."

"You can do this, find your confidence."

"Ticktock, I don't have all day!"

"Do not make them wonder why they are reading my words and not yours."

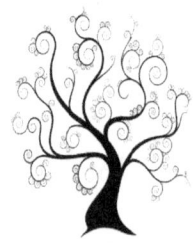

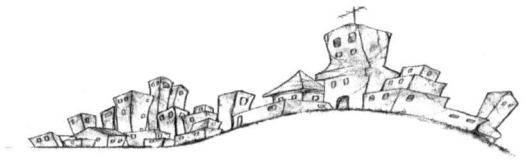

Okay, okay, I got it!

"Confused yet?"

"Welcome to my insanity."

My inner voices tend to speak, and when I say speak, they are usually overbearing and loud. The only way to alleviate the constant internal conflict in my head is to acknowledge their presence.

I have been stigmatized by the human zoo as broken, challenging, and even a burden. The Grim Reaper waits patiently, as he knows insanity is the trick he has imposed for the collection of his souls.

"Would I be considered crazy?"

It is a matter of one's perspective, ultimately.

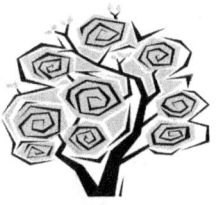

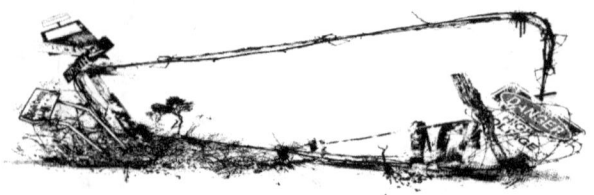

Here is a thought to neutralize the toxic shame when looked upon by others. I could stick a pair of earbuds in my ears and masquerade the voices in my head by giving them names. I assume that would delude some of the curious onlookers. Somehow talking to yourself with earbuds stuck in ones' ears is "normal."

You are going to hear a lot of inner dialogue between myself and the unnamed voices.

When does it stop?

The cells bathe in potent chemicals causing information to misfire in an endless loop. It is an idiopathic race of spontaneous Russian roulette. It draws you in and pushes you out, often simultaneously.

The episodes of depression led to the deliberate precarious behaviour that always resulted in self-harm. I existed only one half of the time.

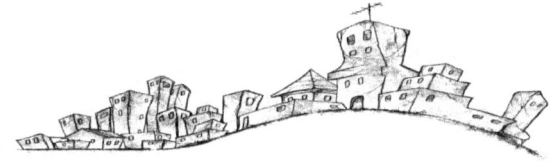

A silent crack from the eggshells that cover the floors triggers an irrational frenzy towards the fearful innocent eyes.

"Stand tall.

Be oblivious to,
Everything and all.

You cracked a shell.
I am far from well.

I will scream,
And I will yell.

I do not know why,
I feel this way.

Lost touch with reality,
On this very day.

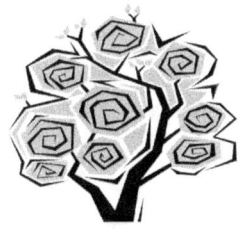

In this state,

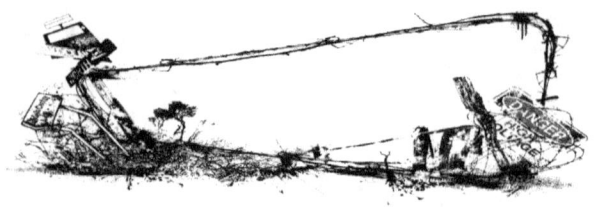

*And in this mind,
Please help,
I need to escape*

*I cannot wait.
Hurry before it's too late!"*

The sound of the roaring sirens is nearing. Time is running out!

The blood-spattered across my wrist is like the reddest most divine of rose petals plucked from its core, slowly descending to the floor. Intrigued by the formation of the masterpiece, I awaited the inquiry and judgement of the mindless collective. It was the formality before the punishment of assimilation. I do not know what I do is wrong, as I am consumed by the evil that Pandora has unleashed upon this world.

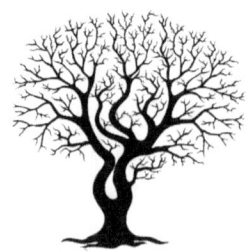

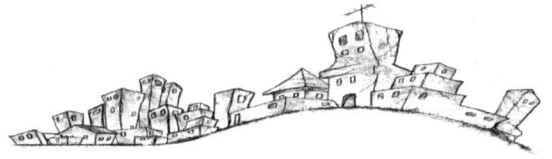

Evil, death, and lost hope blankets my hands as I patiently await the reckoning of the zombie apocalypse. Evil is as evil does, but lost hope can be hope found within Pandora's box.

"The stagnate air holds the whispers ripple hostage,
Repeatedly echoing the stranger's words.

Replicating the internal torture,
Through excreting crimson blood.

Painting a drum that beats onto the tiled floor.

The stranger's taunting whisper,
Accelerating the beating drum.

Rupturing through sound,
Spilling the last of the stranger's words.

The whisper said I must,
Conform."

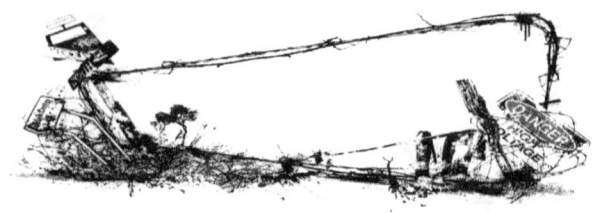

"Disguised, the voices in one's head are mislabeled by society as insanity."

Lori S Moore

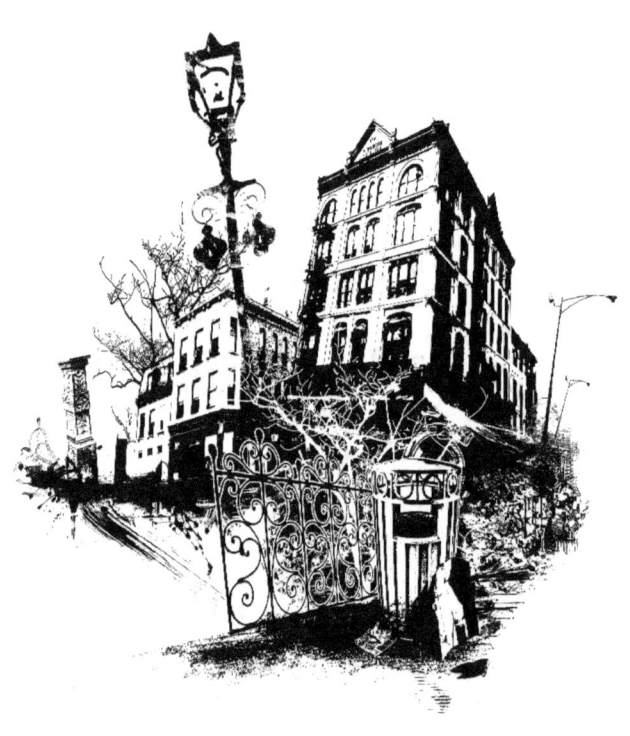

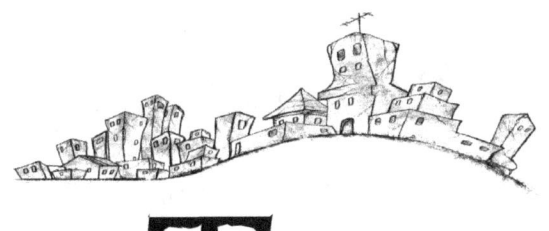

THE PORTAL

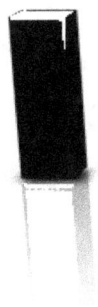

inherited a mind plagued by the complexities of my genetics and environment combined. I was conflicted with the age-old question between nature versus nurture. Which one created the intricate labyrinth inside my head only to forget the map to guide me to reason. Where insanity breeds and continually evolves. You will undoubtedly follow me down the long journey into the rabbit hole.

"Well, here we go."

"Are you ready?"

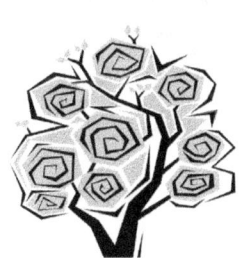

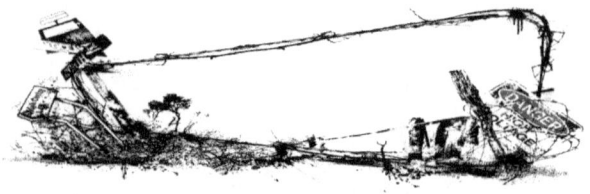

I am drooling waterfalls of exhilaration. I have been waiting for an exceptionally long time for you to see what is in my head. I call it, "Through the Eyes of Insanity."

My mind is like a roller coaster without a functional shut off switch. I am about to give you a once in a lifetime personal guided tour throughout various periods with the hopes of finding out what went wrong.

Now I must ask the big question.

Where and how do I begin?

I am just a girl with a racing mind filled with endless thoughts and imagination. I embrace the flooding of illusions and even a delusion or two that cause my inspirational drowning. Rub the magical lamp, and I will make a wish. Trying to bind my thoughts together in one place would be a great start.

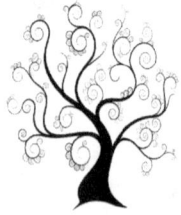

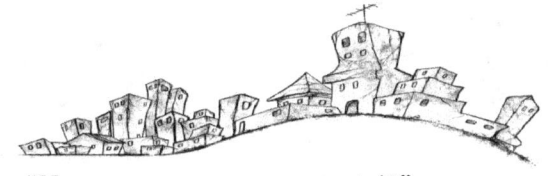

"Have you ever seen a portal?"

A liquified mass that you cannot see through porting you to different places is my definition of a portal. It leaves you tempted to find out what is on the other side.

"Would you agree?"

"Picture the portal in your mind. When you catch a glimpse of the portal in front of you, I will be waiting. It might take a couple of minutes; everyone is different and unique in their response."

"Take a deep breath. I know you can do it, concentrate. I am in no rush and meant what I said. I have been waiting for what seems to be a lifetime to share this with you."

"Now count with me as you inhale through your nose and exhale through your mouth. Relax, you will be in my world soon."

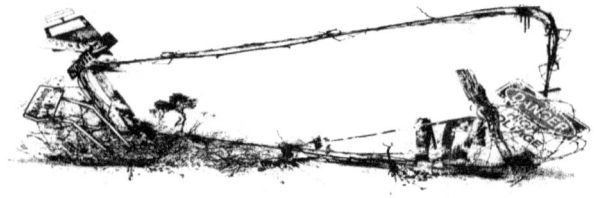

"10 breathe, 9 breathe, 8 breathe…"

"Do you see the portal yet?"

"Keep going, I can barely contain my excitement!"

"7 breathe, 6 breathe…"

"Tell me Mr. Rabbit,
Why do you hop so fast?

Where do you hide?
When your full inside?

Chomping on each blade,
Of the yellow-green grass.

I follow you down,
Into the depths of this hole.

Psychedelically controlled,
My mind is now freed from life's hold.

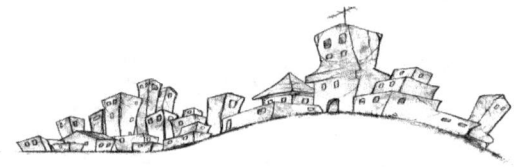

As you turn your head,
And ask me to tea.

An animated bunny,
Now speaking to me.

'Why did Jack and Jill,
He asked,
Tumbledown the hill and crash?'

I paused for a moment,
It lasted forever,
No answer,
No thought.

Then suddenly,
Out came a clock.

With two spinning hands,
Floating through the air.

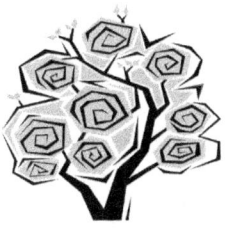

Tick Tock,
Tick Tock,
Bang, Bang,

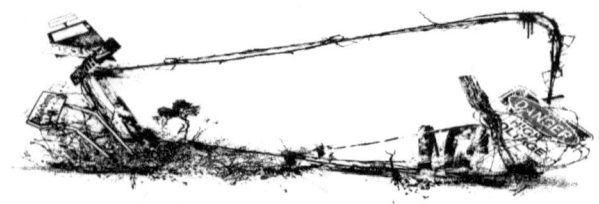

Did you hear the knock?

Coming from the tiny door,
Across the room,
There is a knock.

A voice I hear,
Says come on through.

So, I walked through the door.
I was greeted by a man.

He called himself, Jack,
Then he shook my hand.

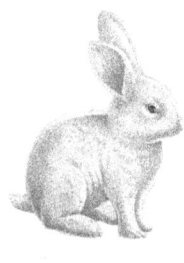

I asked him the question,
The rabbit asked me.

'Mr. Jack,
Why did you tumble,
Down the hill and crash?'

He replied with his eyes,
Gawking at mine.

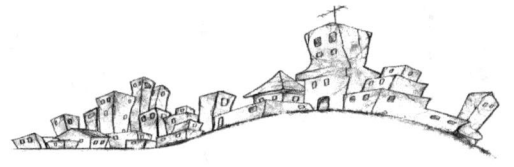

*'My mind has been set free,
Unique and my own.*

*My story has an ending,
You have already known.*

I am not alone,

*I am old,
And I have grown.*

*Tell Mr. Rabbit his answer,
Is all,
But his own.*

*Time is a journey,
Stop,
Breathe,
And look around.*

Listen to the voices.

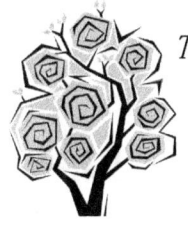

*The stories inside your head.
Inspire your imagination.*

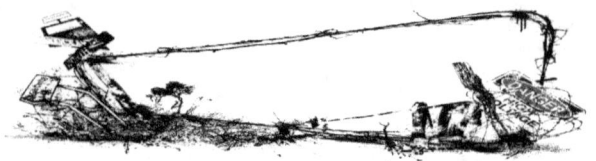

See the colours,
Feel the moment,
Live your dreams.

Escape the depths,
Of the hole you are in.

Open your eyes.
It's a new day to shine.'

Wake up!

Now still as can be,
Chomping on each blade,

The grass both yellow and green.

Is Mr. Rabbit,
Jack,
I will call him by name."

Let the truth be unearthed.

"You made it!"

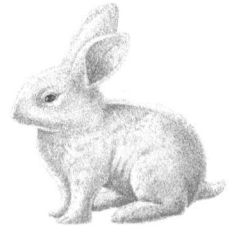

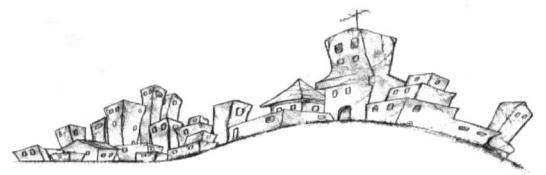

I feel like a nervous child on the first day of school.

The portal is quite extraordinary. I must admit it is mysterious yet has an element of fear but mostly curiosity and intrigue of the unknown. It looks dark and has a circular shape with a liquified center.

"Do you see it now?"

"Are you curious even a little?"

I am going to touch it to see what it feels like.

I am slowly lifting my arm towards it. I cannot stop gazing into the mesmerizing hole of what appears to be nothingness. My hand is almost touching it.

"Take my hand!"

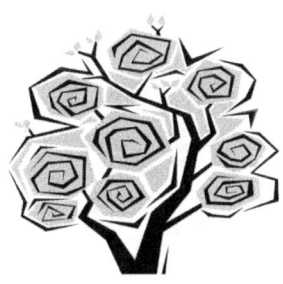

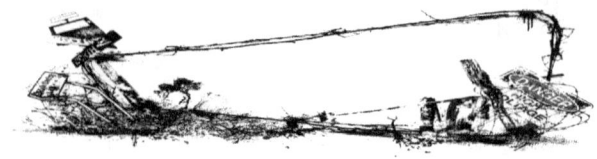

"Ready?"

"1…2…3 go!"

"For only a moment, darkness encompasses this place.

Creating the illusion of confinement,
It is drowning this space.

The eyes are the doorway,
Interconnecting these worlds
One must remain bound to the reality that exists.

To shift the states that I must face.
Inside of the door unraveled desires unhide.

Only to see floating through the air,
each scattered piece fly by.

Drawing me in, I cannot help but to stare.
Flashes of my life rein my flesh beware.

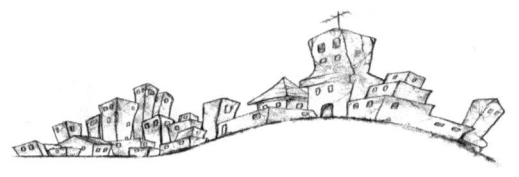

Caught inside an endless loop.

The portal for only a moment,
Encompasses this space."

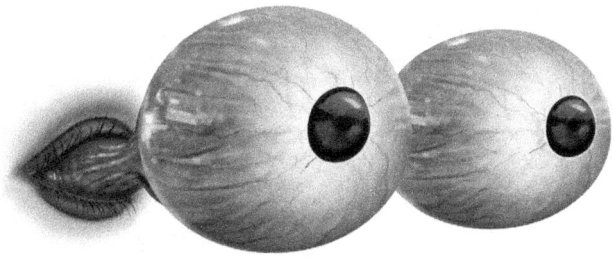

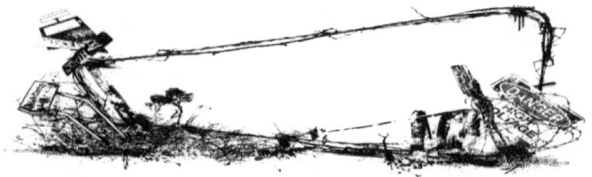

Darkness Falls

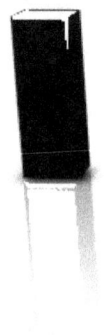 I do not know what happened!

"Watch out there is a wall."

It looks like the brick is crumbling. A picnic table in the middle of nowhere and water; a lake or an ocean. It is endless.

Something is coming. I forgot my glasses. I cannot make it out. It is massive, and it is moving fast. Wait, someone is standing by the water. Whatever is coming this way, it looks to be after whoever is standing there.

It is happening so fast, it is a monster, reptilian possibly. Its mouth is opening.

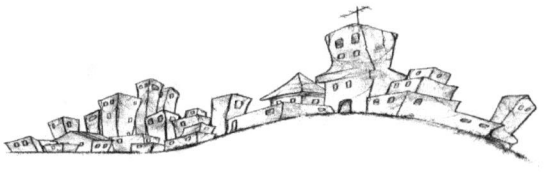

GONE!

"RUN, as fast as you can!"

"Take my hand, the picnic table, jump! Jump as high as you can!"

Whomever that was, they are gone, all in one mouthful.

It is coming for us.

"JUMP!"

"We must go back to the portal. I cannot see it."

"Where did it go?"

"We are trapped!"

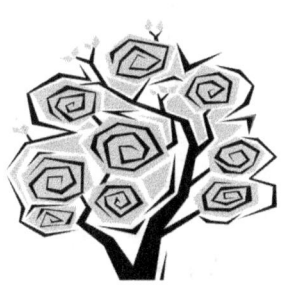

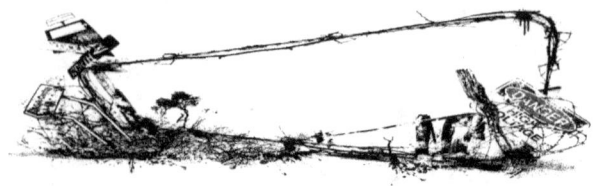

"Imagine yourself being trapped. You cannot move, you cannot even have a coherent thought that makes any sense. You are scared and are alone. You might start to hallucinate; you may also hear things that are not there. You know something is wrong, but you do not know what it is. You cannot ask for help because you cannot explain all the feelings and emotions that are going on inside of you. You are bound by the constant torture of your mind.

You live in fear, and you may even develop certain obsessive behaviours to cope with your fluctuating mind just to ease the pain.

Your sad, and you do not know why but you do know nothing makes you happy even the things you once enjoyed.

You become so withdrawn from society that people make you uneasy, and you fear that they are staring and laughing at you. You cannot walk right because they are watching. You

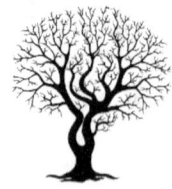

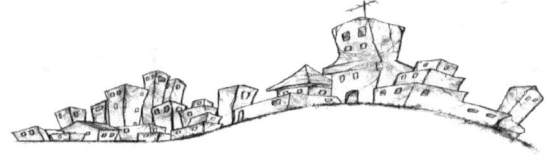

cannot do anything right. You cannot think or breathe.

Suddenly you have a burst of energy, and all you can do is talk and make plans. You are finally confident, and you cannot do anything wrong. You do risky things like spend all your money and make altering life choices.

Then the inevitable happens, you crash.

You slowly crawl back into your corner and wish you would never wake up. The mental and physical pain can sometimes be too much to bear. Consequently, your life cycles in the same pattern repeatedly."

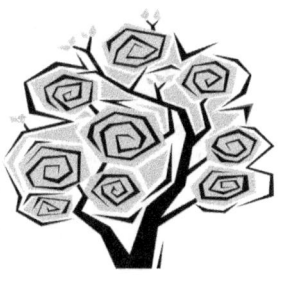

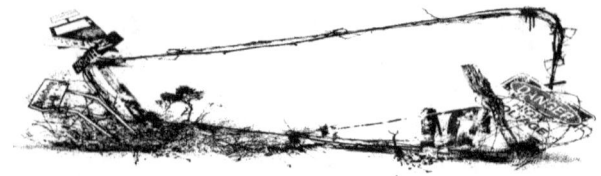

Think!

My mind is the maze, and the labyrinth does not end here.

"Take my hand!"

I know what to do.

"Submerged into the mercy of cruel torment is a human body, both fragile and powerless. The scarlet blood that seamlessly maneuvers throughout each vein and artery has been tainted. The invisible disease slowly breaks down both the body and mind. The soul not affected by the plagues carries the encumbrance of the injustice for the suffering.

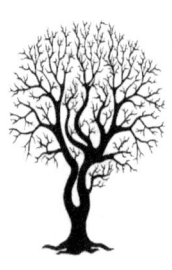

Quiet the voices that mutter to me.

Obtrusive and unrecognizable,
The whispers hidden beneath.

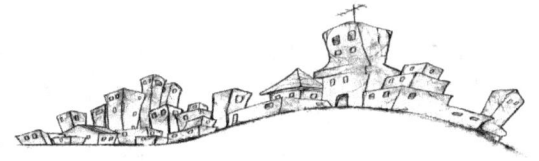

No manifested words to fear.
Silence, I will keep.

I will not spill a sound.

A promise to you,
Ignore and retreat.

The torso quivers from the fire raging inside as it claws its way out of the battlefield. A war that intensifies each time the hand on the clock moves but only a second. The self-destructed mind is now sheltered from the imprinted persecution of the lasting torment of the liquefying body.

How do I elude the contorted death of my time?

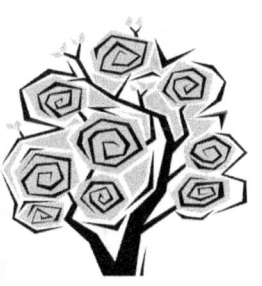

Pulled deep,
Ahold,
Break me free.

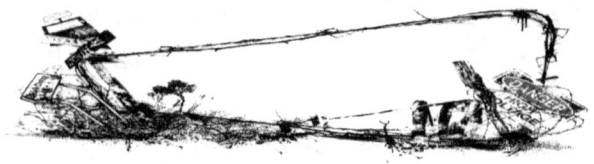

I beg,
I pray,
I choose to live,
Each day,
A life,
My life.

Without warning from the loud and unrecognizable voices, something delicate emerges. The whisper broke free from beneath the chaos.

I ask to be saved.
This heat, I cannot bear it, for one moment longer.

The soft and comforting soul born from my roots emerges.

'I will take your burden. Dream of a place that is safest from all your wounds. Recover it and live in that moment like it is the last moment of your life. I will ease your suffering and secure it all away.

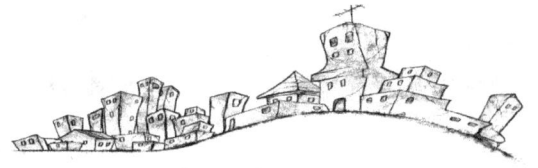

*I am the gateway.
You paid in full.*

*The burden of torment,
I took,
All from you.*

You are free from the fires, the battles, the internal storm that rages within. Rejuvenating are the veins and arteries overflowing with the scarlet blood. Purified from the diseases that spread and cause you your pain.

*I open the gates,
Come take my hand.*

*Shielded and protected,
Back to your place.*

*Your dream,
Your moment,
Safe from this
war.'*

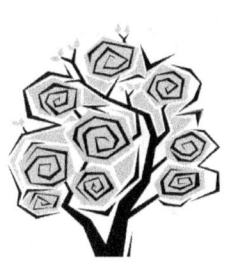

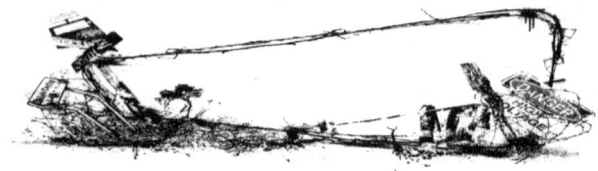

My war,
The war from within."

It is cold!

The temperature is dropping rapidly.

"Can you feel it?"

Suffocation, each breath gets harder to take.

My toes, it is travelling up paralyzing every part of my body. There are no coherent thoughts left.

We are trapped!

There is no light, only darkness wrapping over this entire space.

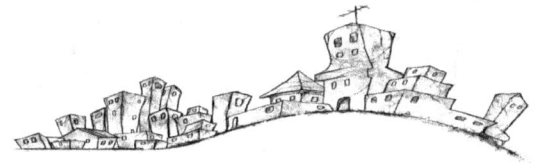

We are bound by the constant torture of my mind. The fear and solitude generate an intense emotional uphill roller coaster ride that we cannot escape from.

> " *The spider whispers psycho,*
> *Spinning crazy thoughts.*
>
> *'Sleep now, my dark angel,*
>
> *Disorientation*
> *Now off your feet.*
>
> *Time will move much slower,*
> *A promise I will keep.'*
>
> *Run,*
> *Crawling closer,*
> *Whispers psycho*
> *Crazy spirals deep.*"

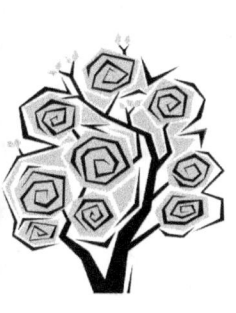

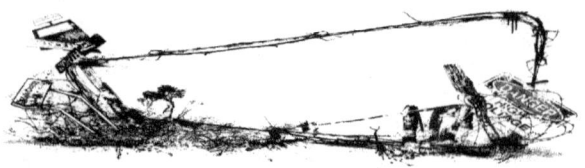

"I am hoping you are ready for the ride."

"What was that?"

" What do you see in the space before your eyes?
The key in disguise?

Light that illuminates darkness,
Darkness in the absence of light.

The mind interprets a limited perception of what can be seen,

Bound by the reality of our existence.

Unseen is the lack of comprehension.
The emptiness,
The nothingness,
The empty spaces of the in-between.

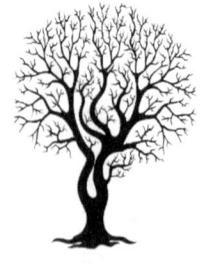

Within earth's heaven and hell,
Not things made up.

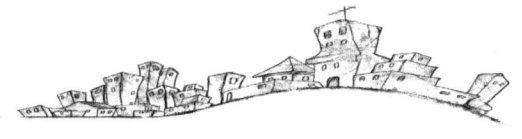

How can nothing be something at all?

The elements combine,
Fused,
Flawed by design.

Evolving the army,
Unravelling the mystery,
Scattered pieces throughout time.

Past, present, and future,
The puzzle defined.

Seek the truth,
All the answers you will find.
Erase what is in your mind.

Unlearn and deprogram,
Forget every thought,
Forget every word.

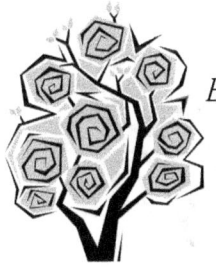

Invoke all senses,
Escape into the journey.

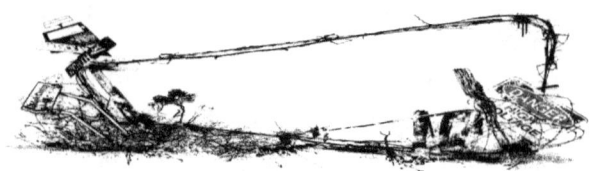

*There is a door,
There is a place,
In a different realm,*

Within the empty space."

Even in darkness, my twisted mind becomes an amazing delusional maze. There is nothing ordinary about the way my mind foresees my past, present and the future.

There is a beginning, a long string of starts without any distinct line of reason. I am not sure when reality becomes a delusion, or is the delusion just part of my existence?

"Are they staring at you yet?"

"Do you feel the eyes on you and that laughter echoing?"

"Did you hear it?"

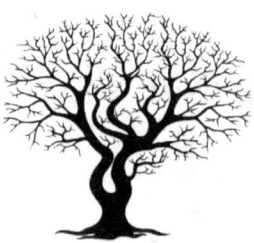

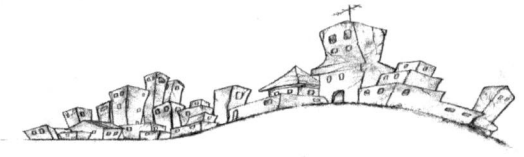

A whisper, it is getting louder. I cannot make it out. It is unsettling, I cannot tell if its real or just a dream.

"How does it make you feel?"

"Can you hear it?"

"Wait!"

"STOP!"

"Look, there is a light just up ahead. We are almost out of the darkness. Stop, just for a moment. I need to breathe. I am about to show you things that I have never shown anyone before."

"Nervous, scared, happy and every emotion in-between is rushing through my body. I need to take a couple of deep breaths. Let us stop for just a moment. Having you here with me is a big step."

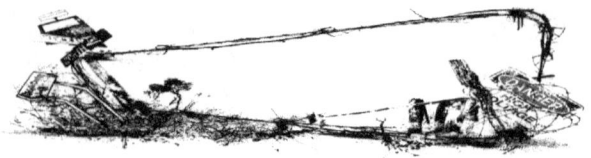

"Get it together already!"

"I am trying, I am trying!"

"Leave me alone!"

"I will find my way; just give me a second."

"They won't wait for you forever; in fact, even I'm getting bored."

"Alright!"

"Get out of my head!"

"Okay, let us go I think I am ready now."

"The image is still somewhat blurry; it reminds me of an old television with rabbit ears that need to be fine-tuned. If we get closer, it might refine itself."

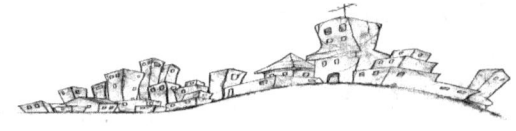

"Ah, there I am."

"Shall we begin?"

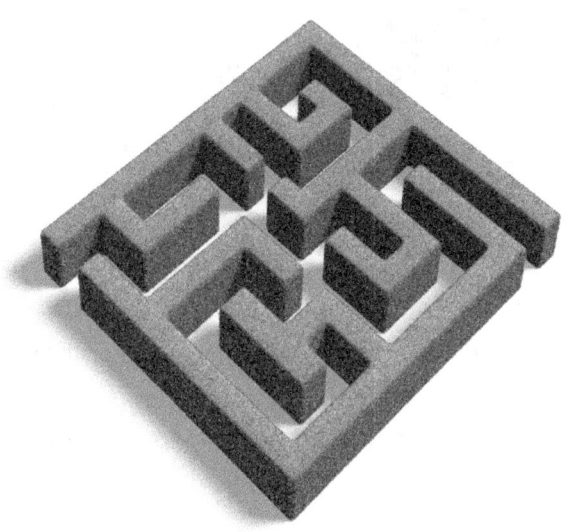

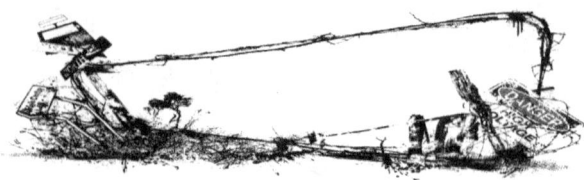

THE ESCAPE

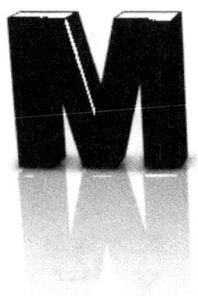y first memory as a child brings me back to my three-wheeler. It was orange, not to fancy. A plain three-wheeled model, so to speak with rust noticeably surfacing through the once shiny painted surface.

"Should I stay or make a run for it?"

I felt desperate that hot summer day. I just had lunch and decided I needed to go outside. I stood on the hard patio stones assessing my surroundings, planning my get-a-way.

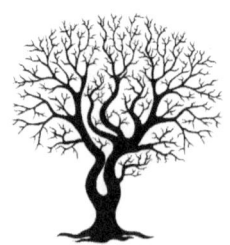

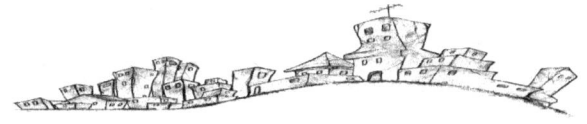

I could see lush green grass, or was it all the unattended weeds exploding between the cracks of the charcoal-coloured stones. In any case, it was ultimately the path that was going to lead me to my freedom.

"What was I running from?"

"Where was I going?"

I was fighting the feeling of tiny black ants climbing up my pale skin scattering throughout my clothes. There were thousands of them marching like a parade at a picnic.

Shivering in disgust, I snapped!

I had to go!

So, I did.

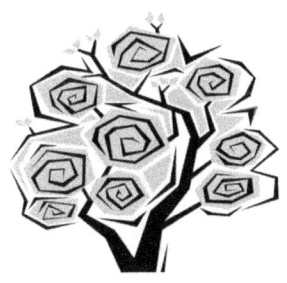

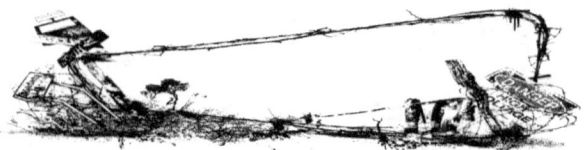

I drove that orange rusted three-wheeled bike as fast as I could peddle with my little feet. I was three, and I had a mission. I believe it was my first of many.

"Where am I?"

"Am I dreaming?"

The dreams and nightmares walk a fine line with reality and often can be confused, especially in the minds of the delusional. Sometimes it is the dreams and nightmares that dominate the hidden truths within us.

"Which is it?"

"How do you know the difference?"

"Truth is sometimes I cannot."

"How do you know the difference between your reality and what you dream of?"

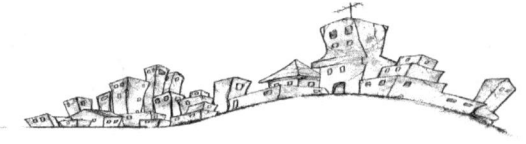

*"There is a line rarely seen,
Drawn by fate,
Controlled by time.*

*Defend oneself instinctually,
To survive the poetic march.*

*The internal savage beats its drum.
A rhythmic beat played by one.*

*Summoned the beast the mind has done.
To shield the battle,
A war they've won."*

"Contemplate for a moment that the worlds and ideas you create inside your mind is the actual reality. In turn, what you call reality is the delusion of your existence."

"Why are we here?"

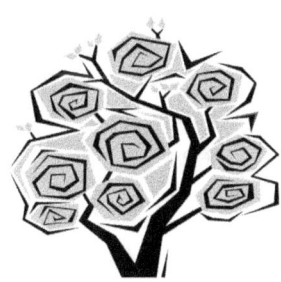

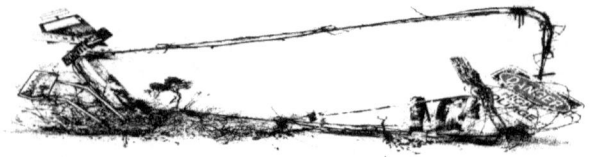

"Who made us?"

The bigger question is the key to the meaning of life.

We often wonder how life began. Were there gods, or just, one god? What about alien life or are there just scientific explanations that are still being calculated and rationalized. Are we an experiment trapped in a world of illusions and hidden dimensions?

"What if life began with not just one of those theories but all of them?"

"What if we are all right on how our existence took shape on some level?"

It would be kind of like pieces to a more giant puzzle. The sane and the insane see the world differently, but maybe it is for a reason.

The problem is complicated, and different minds need to see things that might not otherwise be seen.

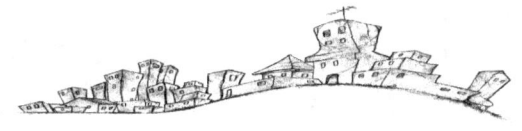

The sheer fact that we cannot agree on how we came into existence could be why we will never figure it out.

Until humanity, one day concedes to the many ideas as being all part of one. Maybe then, the power of many minds could project one idea answering what we have always questioned.

Total unity a concept that humans have never been able to achieve.

Fact or fiction, life and death, the world beyond our own.

"Time, existence, what does this mean to you?"

How does one perceive the world so differently from another?

Who is right?

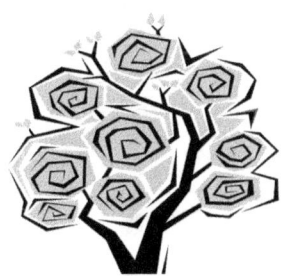

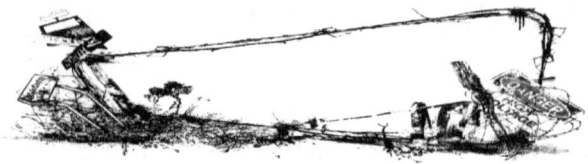

Who is wrong?

Maybe there is no wrong answer. Closed mindedness shelters people from the thoughts that something else out of their belief system could exist. It could essentially turn their world upside down. It could destroy everything they were taught and question their existence and teachings.

The insane see dimensions of life, an existence with no boundaries. Creativity and off the wall ideas are mangled inside the mind. Patiently, waiting to be deciphered and accepted by the sane.

I see things that are not there. Maybe insanity has its perks.

"Look around you right now."

"What do you see?"

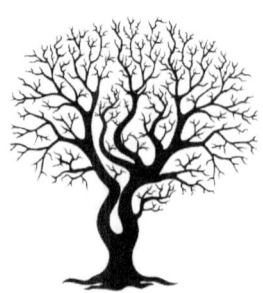

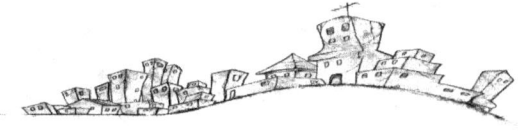

" I am not who you think I am.
I watch the darkness in the light.

Monsters running free,
Staring and watching over me.

This empty shell,
I do not belong here.

Save me,
Set me free."

You probably see the things that are obvious and right in front of you. The items you can touch and feel.

Do you see the wind as it blows?

What if there are things in the room other than what you can feel and touch?

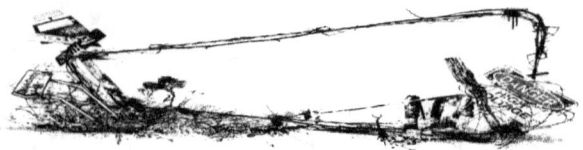

We look directly at the objects in front of us but ignore the empty spaces.

What if they were not empty spaces?

We have been trained to ignore the things that do not activate our senses. When I look around, I do not just see the window with the grey curtains hanging from them. I see much more.

How?

Space is never empty. It is just our mind that perceives it that way.

Puzzle pieces are floating throughout the air if I could just grab one. Each piece represents a memory that holds the key to the completed picture. If I could just reach one.

"Wait, you have one?"

"What is it?"

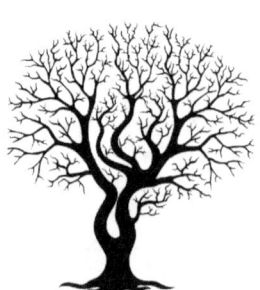

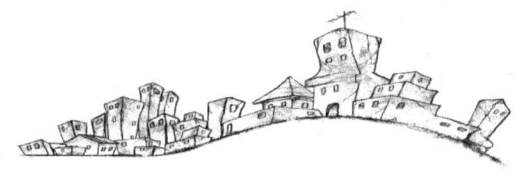

"To be extraordinary is to conceive that the mind is unique."

- Lori S Moore

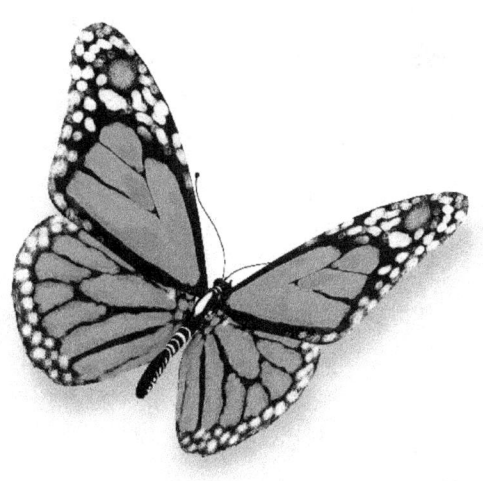

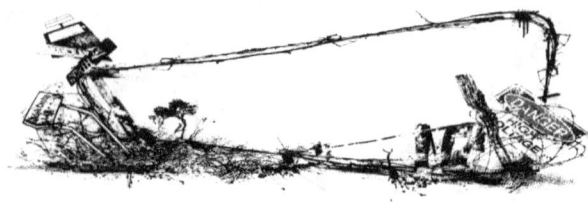

R*EJECTED*

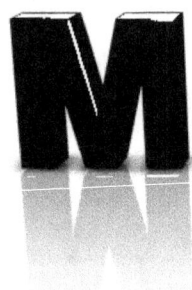y mother, a woman continuously challenged both mentally and physically, lacked necessary nurturing skills. The age-old question was her affliction, a case of nature versus nurture.

She grew up in a household where showing someone that you loved them did not exist. A simple hug and I love you was impossible to conceive. This, combined with flawed family genetics, was just the beginning of her detrimental plight, and mine.

I was assembled in avocado green polyester pants and a mustard yellow t-shirt.

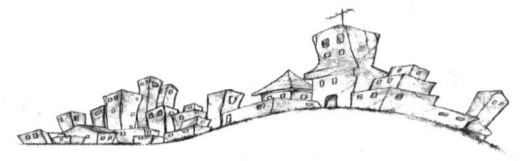

It was my first day of junior kindergarten, and I was already an outcast. You would have thought that the long tail dragging on the floor behind me was real. In some cultures, green symbolizes peace and safety, and yellow as caution.

If I had to interpret the message of how I looked and felt that day, it would be described as a four-year-old plagued by emotional chaos. My trembling limbs tell me to take a step forward, but my mind says proceed only with your eyes wide open.

"You are not like them."

It was not just the clothes that set me apart from the others that I imagined were monsters. I believed it could have been my lack of social skills and refusal to conform to a single box. I learned at a noticeably young age that I was different. I was a mixed-up child; naturally, that was the good news.

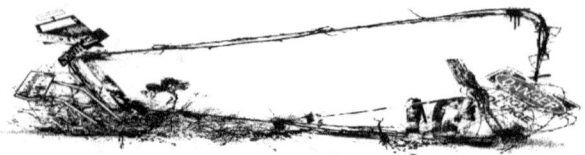

I was rejected by most people as plain weird. Who would have thought that I was that strange kid wrapped around a tree begging for someone to befriend me or even pretend they liked me.

Jack and Jill or Mr. Mugs, that was the determining factor of your initial social status. The smart kids belonged to Mr. Mugs, and the intellectually challenged were Jack and Jill. Give you one guess what group I belonged to. Maybe it makes sense. My intellect is somewhat limited to the mental capacities of a crazy person, one who obsesses, for example, with post-apocalyptic movies.

In the present day, I sometimes wish the overpopulated world would perish. I contemplate zombies or a lethal virus. A plague that spreads viral, bacterial, fungal, parasitic, maybe even a bioweapon.

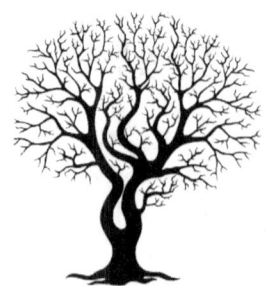

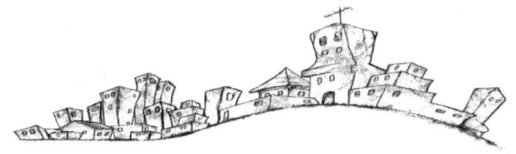

The immunocompromised and much of the healthy succumb to the sickness, and humanity falls to only a handful.

I fantasize about simplicity without resistance and lesser changes. I do not mind being alone as I rule the world in my solitude. The thought of it is exhilarating. I can feel a tiny smirk emerging, oh how I wish I could be a vampire and live forever in this world I have created. I would not fear disappointment from others and its never-ending torment. The race inside my mind never ends, I remember the start, but I cannot seem to find the finish line.

The children who were monsters lived under the floor and dug their tunnels attached to the city sewers, patiently waiting for their next victim.

Vicious and bloodthirsty, they follow your scent while plotting the next attack. The flesh will be ripped and consumed while the bones scattered across the wasteland, they call home.

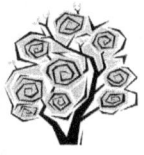

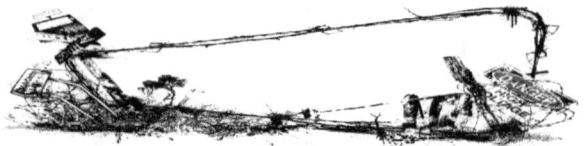

The stale smoke in the basement lingered in the air each time I reluctantly slithered down those stairs. Cold and dark when alone, full of fear in the room that seems unknown.

"The light, the light, why won't you turn on?"

The darkness begins to fade as the glowing amber light engulfs the blackened room. Conceived by two but born from one, dark to light and back to dark. The innocence that forms disappears from the world I call home. The integrity born to me has now but gone, stolen, and destroyed by the monsters that roam. I have been followed; I am not safe; they caught my scent.

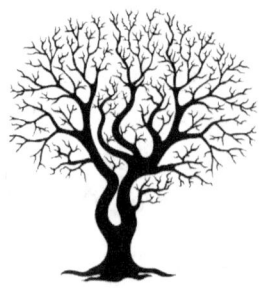

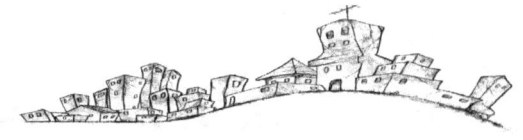

*"Cold as ice, I'm frozen in fear.
Stuck to its block as I wait till the thaw.*

*The monsters have retreated to their tunnels,
through the sewers, back to their home.
The wasteland with bones.*

*I fear they will return, so I am always on guard.
Waiting for my blood to spatter the walls.*

*I envision them returning to the hell in which they came,
But not before being dragged back as their trophy of bones."*

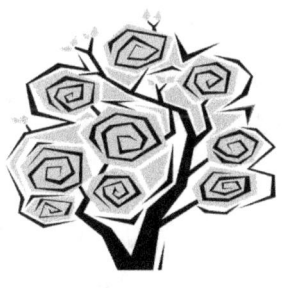

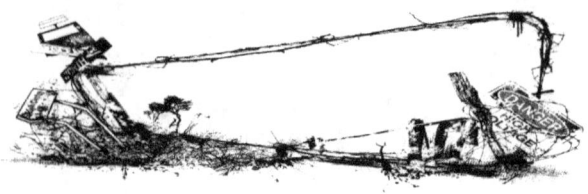

THE BLUE RUBBER RING

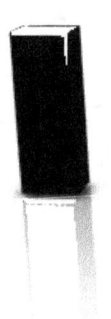

It starts with a grain of sand.

I imagine myself in a dark room, my hands are out with my palms facing up. In my hands, a grain of sand rests. Right now, it is just that, a very tiny grain of sand, a dark spec with brownish tones nothing more.

Or is it?

Maybe I should look again.

I close my eyes for ten seconds while slowly inhaling from my nose and exhaling from my mouth.

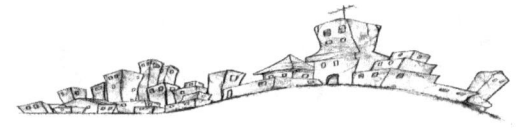

...10 breathe, 9 breathe, 8 breathe...

A liquified gateway rippled and slightly distorted; I stood perplexed, gazing without any movement. Once processed, I lifted one hand with my index finger curiously and cautiously, contemplating making my way through.

There is a strange blue rubber ring on the bathroom door. I was told that was how you knew the bathroom was in use as a four-year-old was not allowed to have locked doors. That was the first thing I saw when entering this new school from the outside doors of the kindergarten classroom. There were double hooks and benches for our school bags and coats, but I noticed the small bathroom and that blue rubber ring foremost.

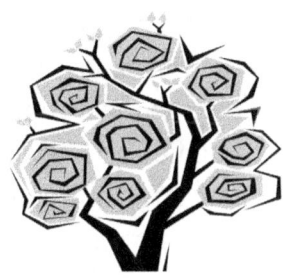

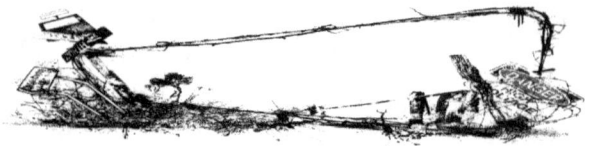

My head turned back to the liquified gateway as I contemplated and silently panicked inside. There is no going back. Life starts to move you forward, not even the delusional world you create can stop the hands of time from proceeding.

A deep breath I must take, one foot in front of the other and move. Where else are you going to go? You have nowhere to hide, nowhere to run. Look, and pay attention.

There was a sandbox and a water station to the left and a long line of cupboards wall to wall with sliding doors. Above the cabinets were oversized windows with sights of the entire schoolyard. The interior of the room to the left was my teacher's desk, Miss Mei was her name.

The most memorable words that rolled off her tongue was the desire to preserve her students in the cupboards that lined the left wall. She wished we would stay these small beings endlessly. I have never forgotten those words as bizarre, as locking someone in a cupboard for eternity may sound.

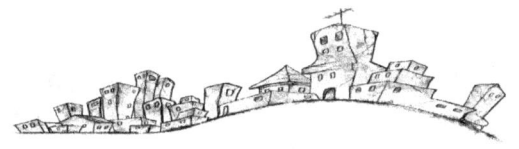

I stand in this peculiar spotlight, but there is also something else that surrounds the outside of this light. It is dark, midnight black with a consistency resembling tar coating and adhering to everything it touches. A distorted hand begins to reach out, just brushing the edge of the light. My eyes continuously attempt to focus, but I cannot see beyond the glow. I am surrounded as I turn rapidly in a circle.

"Welcome to the madness,
Imprisoned within these walls.

Come closer to the chaos,
Infect their only souls.

I hunger for the madness,
Make them all insane.

Degrade them into nothing,
I will use them all the same."

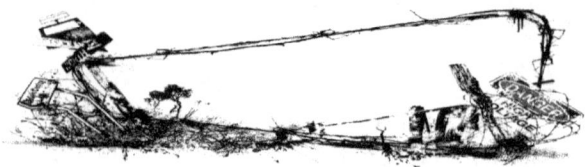

I should scream! I need to cry, but I am frozen and paralyzed at what I cannot fully see.

*"Run with me.
Take me away from all this insanity.*

*Hear the voices whispering to me.
Run with me, set me free."*

Close your eyes, close your eyes!

*"The kingdom gates are open.
Come join me and be my slave.*

*Tortured and abused,
Gutted from the brain.*

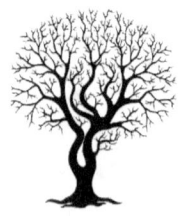

*I will steal all humanity,
A monster you will become.*

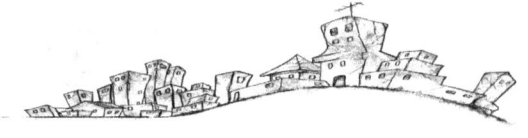

> *Lost in my madness,*
> *I've got you one by one."*

Look at me, love me, hold me.

> *"No more dreams of freedom,*
> *My will and hope have gone.*
>
> *Plagued diseased and broken,*
> *Who have I become?*
>
> *Look into the mirror,*
> *It reveals the truth to see.*
>
> *I am not who I was before,*
> *Transformed and imprisoned*
> *Inside the madness,*
> *Trapped inside these walls.*
>
> *Shattering the mirror,*
> *Fractured is each piece.*

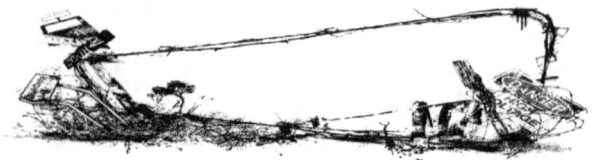

The truth revealed is real insight.

Bleeding bloody hemorrhaging,
Spreading to the rest.

Expose the light a glimpse you will see.
Cease the madness and control the spread.

Restrict your mind to suppress the rest.
Uncover the shard that holds the key.

Hidden in a pile,
Of all the shattered glass."

Affection and attention, it is that simple. My mental wires are crossed and now and then short out, resulting in a misfire. The sparks do not always ignite like they should. My perception is just that, it is my perception. I do not even know if it is real or my misconceptions.

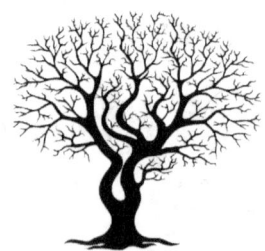

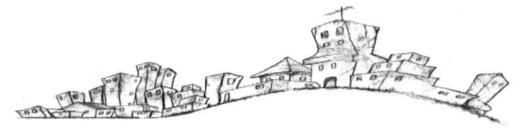

When I ran away on my orange three-wheeled tricycle, I was not running away. I was running towards something, my grandmother, my Meme. She gave me an abundance of love and attention as I was the primary grandchild, her baby girl.

I was her repentance, her do-over. She once told me it was her second chance for the mistakes she made with her children.

Her mistakes affected her seven children very differently. There are four girls and three boys. Each one of them has their own stories and memories, ultimately perceiving their childhood memories from a different viewpoint. Some have pain that lingers consistently, resulting in hidden torment deep inside and unseen to the strangers and even the family that surrounds them. Some have preserved and achieved forgiveness, breaking the dreaded family cycle of emotional neglect.

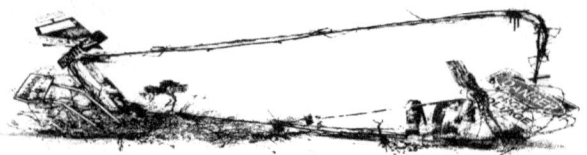

Lastly, the unfortunate ones were plagued with much more than just the family cycle, they inherited the flawed genetics of mental health as well.

"Can you see dead people?"

"Can you see the future?"

I can see into an individual's soul recognizing hidden truths and personal afflictions. I observe people and listen very intently to their stories and comments.

People are like puzzles.

Distinguishing how to fit the pieces together comes from understanding the concealed meanings and hidden truths to get the completed puzzle.

Things can be hidden away and never seen by the average person on the outside.

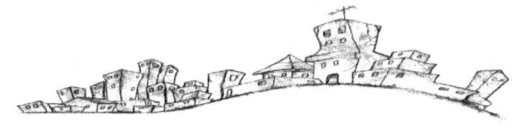

The cupboard of Miss Mei was a place that symbolized affection. The most significant encouraging memory of age four.

In front of the room, a large chalkboard covered in numbers, and the alphabet plastered the wall. In front of the giant chalkboard was an exposed carpeted area where we sat cross-legged and had our nap time. The door that exited the classroom and into the halls of this new room was on the right. Behind our carpeted sitting area were several small tables and chairs where we sat and coloured and drew our stick people.

There was a strange loud bell that rang, leaving remnants of constant vibrations within my ears.

Recess!

I dreaded this time of day not just in kindergarten but every year after that. I walked and paced the schoolyard, mostly alone.

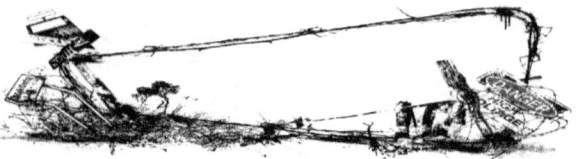

I always questioned if people were staring and talking about me. I could not understand why the connections that most kids made so quickly with each other remained an almost impractical milestone in my case.

The same loud bell sounds once more endlessly imprinted within my head. Out of the spotlight and back into the room, the blue rubber ring sits on the doorknob once again. The liquified gateway through the ripples I see, stepping backwards, I make my way through.

...3 breathe, 2 breathe, 1 breathe...

Open your eyes.

Now look again.

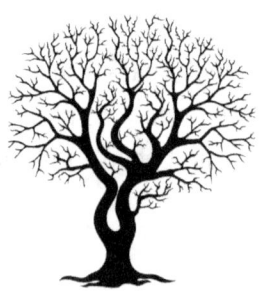

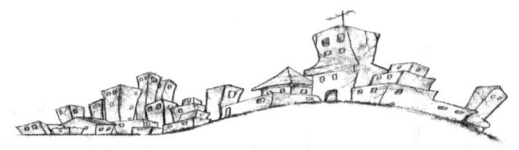

I shift my eyes downwards, trying to focus beyond the darkness. The tiny grain of sand that still sits in the palm of my hands has begun to change. Slowly I watch this microscopic grain of sand begin to illuminate, creating a shift in what I once perceived as only darkness and loneliness.

The light may be small, but things can evolve and grow if we choose to let it.

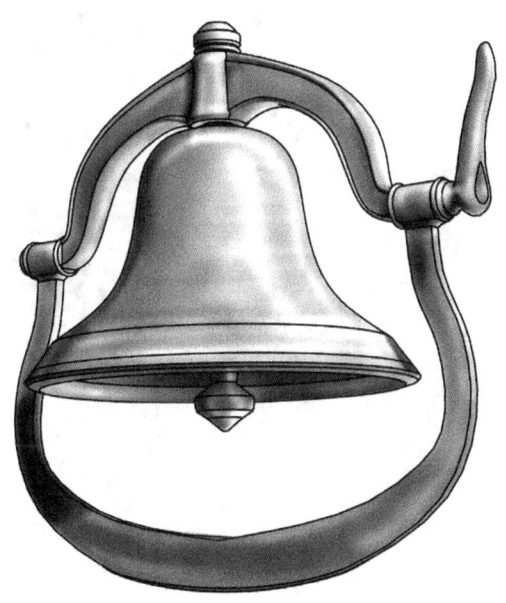

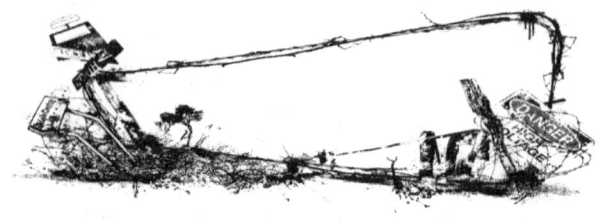

"There is no hope if one forgets to dream."

- Lori S Moore

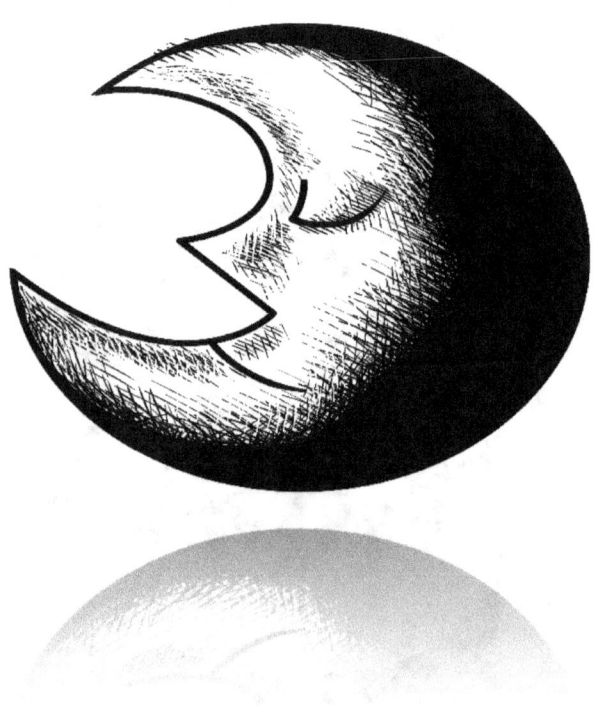

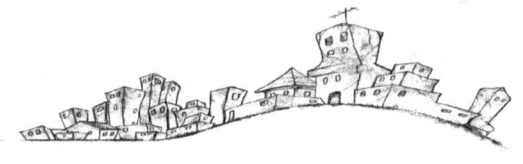

Walking the Rope

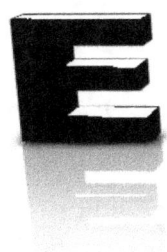

"Ever look at a door and wonder what is on the other side?"

I speak about a glimmer of hope. The thin rope must be balanced upon and walked across to achieve this mission. The light remains soft and dim with shadows of dancing memories projecting on the cave-like walls. Underneath the thin braided rope is a void, a limbo, and a black hole combined. It waits to swallow everything in its reach.

The circus is in town, and we are the star attraction.

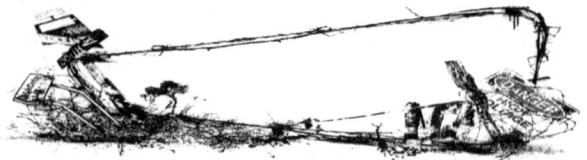

The idea of having to walk this rope is terrifying. One wrong move, and it is over. I stand idly staring at the twine, knowing we must get to the other side like the chicken crossing the road in a child's first joke.

Why did the chicken need to cross the road in the first place? Did the chicken need to get to the other side?

In any case, life requires taking steps that may not want to be walked to move forward.

The first step is the hardest as breathing becomes laboured, and droplets of perspiration begin to moisten my body.

The ringmaster sits between the clowns with the cherry red noses and colourful puffy silk costumes. He anticipates the commencement of the audition.

Then I hear it.

"Ladies and gentlemen, boys and girls, children of all ages," it is time.

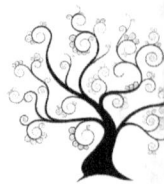

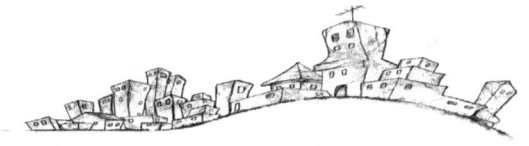

The perspiration is now drenching my body.

I heard the doctor tell him he has two weeks to live. The tears flooded my eyes as I stood against the wall in the hallway next to his room. I repeatedly questioned what I had heard as I became weaker with disbelief, slowly sliding down the wall until I hit the floor.

> *"Absolution is the nightmare,*
> *Casting the shadows*
> *Ending time from this space.*
>
> *Flooded comes the memories,*
> *Scattered and out of place.*
>
> *Broken is a fragile mind,*
> *Empty and alone.*
>
> *Jargoned scrambled is each piece.*
> *Blinded blurred and incomplete.*
> *Resonating through each ear,*

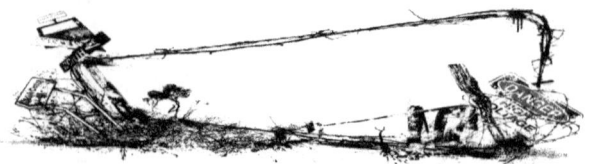

An unknown language speaks unclear.

*Yearning for just one word,
To make it all complete.*

*Shortened is the past,
Hanging onto one last breath.*

*Piece by piece I see a face,
Clearer it becomes.*

*The reaper sits alongside his bed,
and says:*

*'Take my hand, your breath is gone.
The life you had is now your past.
You lived your life but now*

You're dead.'"

We are born, we live, and we die.

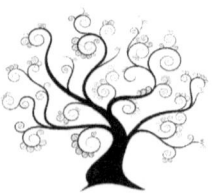

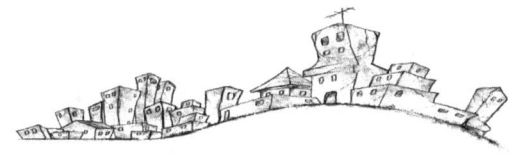

Being born was our parents' choice. Our lives and what we do with it is our choice, but death is always inevitable. No one can predict when that time will come.

"What if today was your last day on earth, what would you do?"

Unless faced with that terrifying notion, how could anyone honestly answer that question to any degree?

The rope in front of us represents both life and death. Successfully crossing the line continues our journey but one false move, and we become lost in the black hole swallowed by the unknowns of the void.

"Is it worth the risk?"

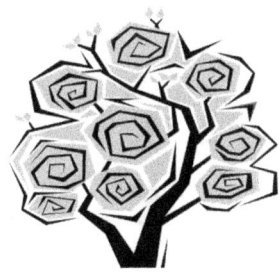

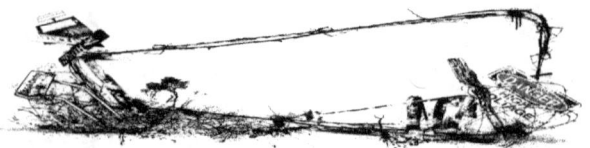

I am imagining myself as a cartoon character visibly seeing my heart popping out of my chest- beating to an irregular rhythm. The feeling of doom intensifies as the dread draws closer. I think I am dying, panic and overwhelming emotions flood through my veins like ice slowly freezing the water of a lake.

"Are you going to cross the damn rope or contemplate life all day?"

Anxiety becomes heavier the longer we carry it within us.

"Let's get this done, we need to move forward."

Hesitantly, I lifted my right foot only to freeze for a moment to catch my breath.

Well, that was not so bad, I can do this!

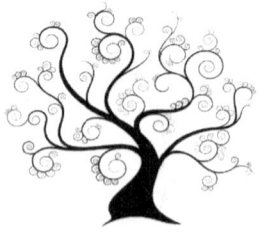

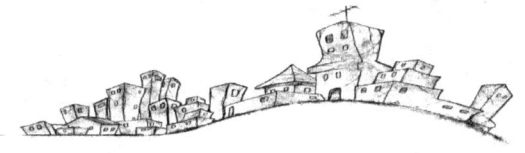

I slowly move my left foot in front of my right and continue each step with more confidence. I am halfway across.

"Are you with me?"

"How are you doing?"

"We are almost there."

"I cannot see anymore what is happening?"

"Have you ever jumped off a plane and waited in anticipation while in free fall to pull the cord on the parachute?"

I have not, but somehow, I envision free-falling each day without a parachute to save me from the dreaded limbo.

Swallowed into the darkness of the void created from the limbo of life.

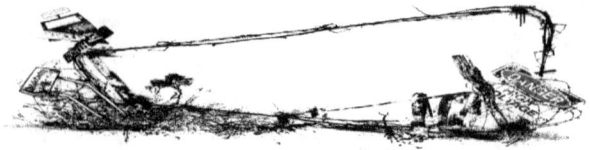

"Do you have a place where you feel safe?"

I have learned over the years that safe areas are not always secure. When we immerse ourselves in these places, we are often alone, and when we are alone, that is when the darkness awakens. Memories become conflicted and shift between good and evil. It overpowers the mind creating delusional thoughts that mask the reason why you hid from the world in the first place.

Mental barriers are the safety switches created within the mind to stop the perception of falling or merely failing. Moving forward and taking chances in life becomes almost impossible when the switches malfunction.

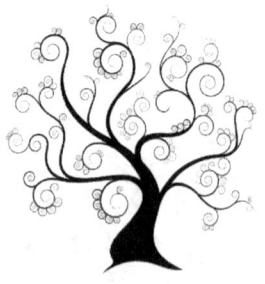

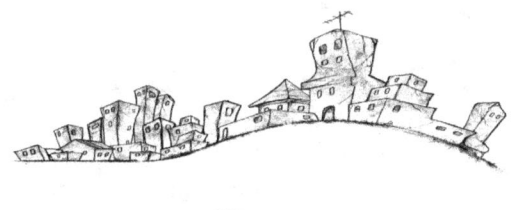

CHOICES

"When you look in the mirror, what do you see?"

I see an image of a woman that still fights to be a little girl. Fear of getting older as each new wrinkle appears on the thickened ageing skin reflected to be my own. The childish mind does not match what is seen in the mirror.

I wish I were a vampire to live through the centuries unscathed, bearing witness to the rise and fall of man. Untouched and preserved, cheating the inevitable death sentence we all are doomed to face. Invincible to wars, sicknesses, and emotions.

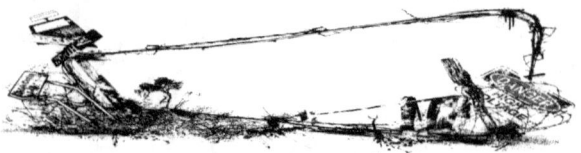

Human emotion is what makes us human, but it is also our weakness. I build walls to protect myself from emotions such as love, hate, fear and happiness. Blocking out these emotions ensures that I do not inflict further pain upon myself at any given time.

If you genuinely love something, you make sacrifices no matter how much you may get hurt in the end. The saying holds for love that is reciprocated; it will return. True love is about sacrificing a piece of yourself for the one you love. Except, I saw it as a motive to get what I wanted. I once made that sacrifice for love, only, I am not sure if it was a selfless or selfish act. I still struggle with that choice I made two decades ago.

I had seen her face for the first time and was confused about how I truly felt inside. Only a monster rejects her flesh and blood, but that is how I felt, and I could not change how she made me feel. I desperately searched for the love I was supposed to feel, but I could not feel it. I did not realize at the time that postpartum depression was the monster that drove this

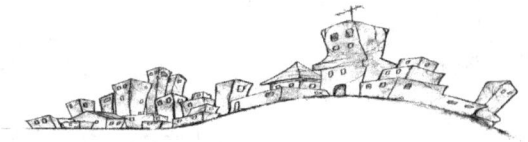

emotionless body closer to the grim reaper. It ultimately became the trigger that escalated by mental breakdowns and future suicide attempts.

Trauma often opens the door to hidden illnesses letting them rear their ugly head in hopes that it can take hold without any resistance. Much like an attack on a weakened immune system. When you get sick, your immune system begins to fight a battle, but those efforts come at a cost. Your immune system starts to weaken, and if exposed to other illnesses, you are at a much higher risk for a war. I believe the same holds true of the mind.

The escalation of the spiral consumed my sadness and drove me into a place where I could not come back from.

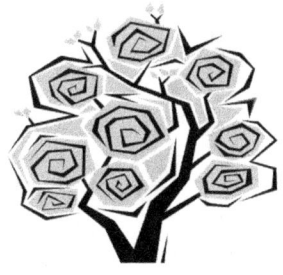

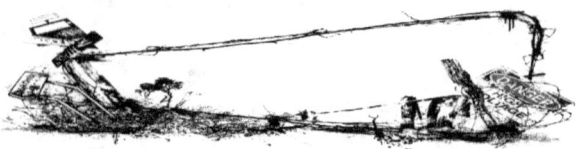

The song at the club as I walked through the doors was what my life became. Pretending that I belonged in a world that could not understand who I was inside was the path I chose. I stood at the crossroads of life, not knowing where each path would lead. There were no signs to aid my decision, only the internal pain and voices telling me I had to make a choice.

"What life do you want to live?"

"Who do you want to be?"

The choice I made has led me to this very moment in my life as I write these words. There are always going to be positive and negative moments in one's life, but my choices had severe consequences that still haunt me to this day.

I lost a piece of myself that day doubting recovery could ever be possible. So now, I wait until the angel of death comes to yield the broken essence of my humanity.

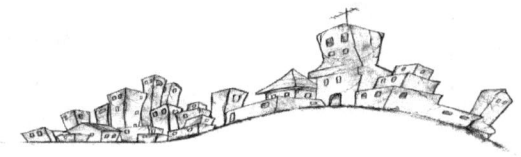

"What if the broken essence of our humanity can be salvaged and saved?"

Not all the soul can be damaged and broken.

What if the right parts are taken and recycled and reused? In each new life that is born to this world.

At birth, we receive our soul, and at death, we give it back so another child can reuse that same soul. Round and round, the experiment of humanity continues.

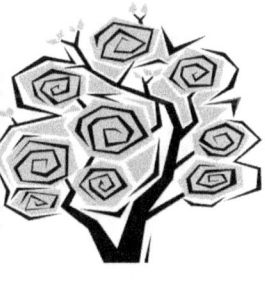

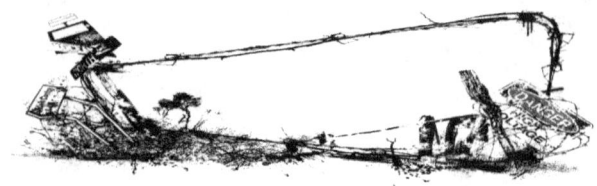

"You must live the past to see the future."
  - Lori S Moore

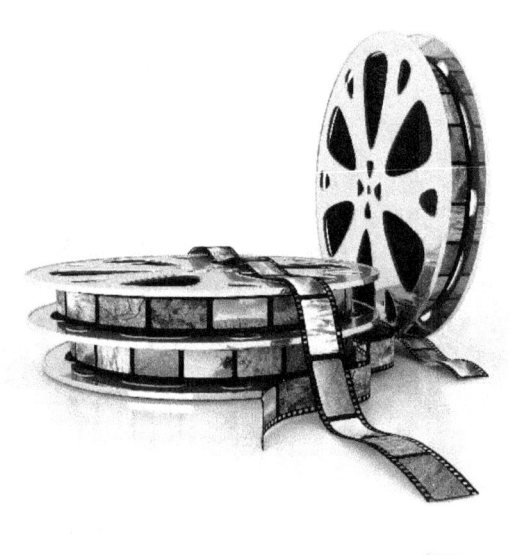

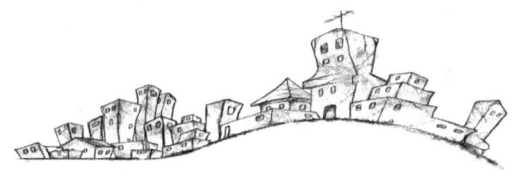

Labeled

"Have you ever washed an article of clothing by hand?"

Once washed, you just wring it out to get rid of the excess water for it to dry. You grip the article of clothing tightly with your hands twisting and squeezing until your hands start to burn and blister.

The twisting and squeezing, coupled with pain, is how I feel inside always when faced with what I did at the crossroads that day. I will die with that pain because forgiveness can never be given to someone that has destroyed the lives of their children. I have given my pound of flesh for the music that still plays in my head from the clubs.

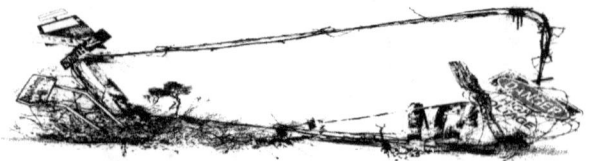

My eyes start to swell and fill with tears even to this day. There is no place beyond the pearly white gates for someone who abandons their child.

The flashbacks of blood dripping from my wrists and countless relationship failures fill the dark void. Hungry and waiting, the void consumes every part of my life where I have done something wrong.

The invisible parachute that malfunctions, as I fall, cannot save me from what I created on my own.

I am worthless and cold lacking real judgement and believe the endless downward spirals in my life are my punishment for my decisions.

My punishment was revealed in my first counselling session when I tried to explain that I feel intense emotions. Not only do I sense my own feelings, but I also absorb the sensations of others around me. The intensity is almost debilitating at times. I do not know how to

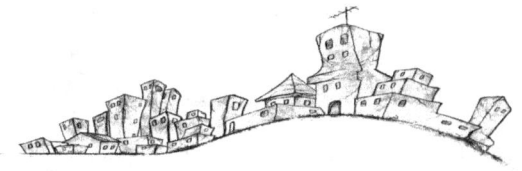

regulate my own emotions, but I can feel the feelings of others to the point of pure pain.

She told me I was an empath.

Perplexed by yet another label bestowed upon myself, I researched what it was to be an empath. I could feel other people's emotions as my own but could not regulate or distinguish which broken emotions belong to who.

It is my superpower, but it is also my punishment for not being able to regulate and understand my own emotions and wrongdoings.

What does it mean to be an empath?

Who am I?

If I was ever lost before, I am surely lost now in this labyrinth of life.

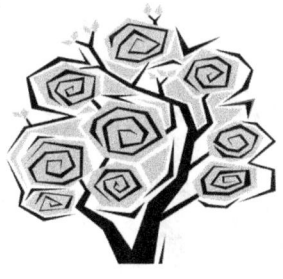

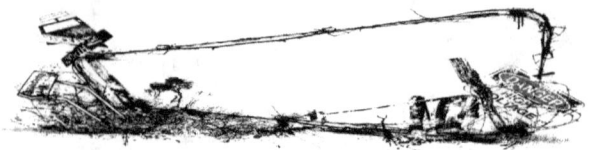

ADHD, Bipolar Disorder, Social Anxiety, Generalized Anxiety, Personality disorders such as Paranoid, Borderline, and Obsessive-Compulsive traits. These are my labels; some have changed, and others have remained over the years.

My labels are just that, labels, but they tell me that I need constant monitoring and help because, within all those labels, suicidal thoughts still emerge. The sadness can be overbearing, and the knife that sits on the kitchen counter tells me, "It can be all over if you pick me up and just do it."

Every day is a fight.

Every day I struggle to keep breathing.

Every day I must remind myself that the next day will come and it will be better.

Every day I must live with my labels and what they mean.

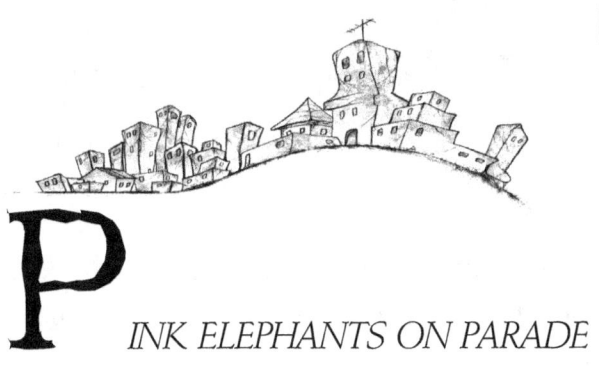

PINK ELEPHANTS ON PARADE

To write coherently requires a state of mind that I have not yet grasped unmedicated. The innuendoes that nurse my words converses in gibberish. An interpretation near impossible and unreliable to make. There is no immunity from the interlocking chains that bind my mind. Chaos, in its pure form, bores the pathways that keep the doors locked until a catalyst finds a way to sneak past.

A silent explosion manifests, triggering the light bulb that activates inside my head. The memories provoked into awakening the fire materializes the perfect parade of smoke, revealing what was once hidden. I gasp for air as

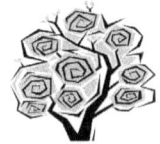

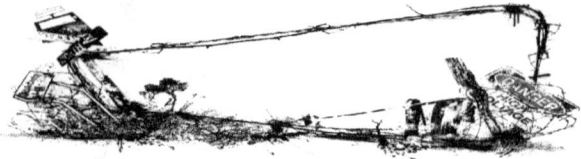

it constricts my lungs suffocating my brain till I vomit the words.

Knock, and the door will open just long enough to catch a glimpse of what will come next.

"Visualize what I am about to say."

The pink elephants have begun their ascension emerging from the stacks of the distant rooftops. The bizarre symphonic harmony plays from the silent radio. Perplexed but curious none the less, my ears fill with the oddity of resonating yodels. The flock of birds effortlessly glide through the breeze in the open sky above.

"Why do the birds speak in complicated riddles through jumbled sound?"

A message, perhaps?

I walked through the door into the crowded room. Led by the spider followed the rabbit, fox, and hound. Outer worldly and appearing translucent in form. These creatures roam freely within the space I called my own. I closed my

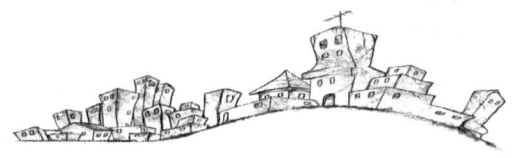

eyes in hopes these animals were all just a crazy dream. I took another breath as I sat with my legs, crossed on my bed. I slowly opened my eyes to hear the spider's words, "Welcome to your chemical nightmare." I watch the alien zoo as the pink elephants' march to an unfamiliar tune, through my room like a parade in the circus of doom.

The spider crept silently behind my heavy staggered footsteps. I made it to the outside steps and sat down for a cigarette break. It was not until I lit my cigarette that the spider revealed itself on the burnt orange brick on the wall of the garage.

The spider was comfortable in the web that stretched from the outside door to what looked like and endless silky scarf floating through the air. It reminded me of a magical carpet ride with exploding retro colours in 3D.

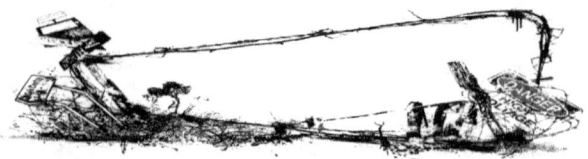

I cannot seem to get used to animals speaking and in English, on top of that. I just kept shaking my head and opening and closing my eyes, but it did not matter. The spider was still waiting for me to accept what was in front of my eyes.

What could a spider possibly have to say as I laughed it off?

Then the unthinkable happened, it spoke.

"As unique is your mind
So is the knowledge you keep
Refined by formal education
Societies normality you seek.

We dumb you down,
And maintain all control.
Comprehend all languages.
We learnt to speak, read, and write.

Know the place that you came from,
All countries, continents, and lakes.

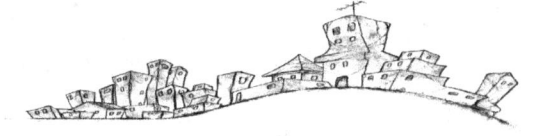

Computed complex mathematical calculations,
The solutions you will not find.

Remember the blood that spilt to the floor.
The villains and heroes who fought in the war.

We developed the super army.
Disguised in human flesh.

Follow the trail,
Of the intricate weave.

I told what was classified,
But you will not recall.
Stay dormant,
And wait to be summoned.

Asleep concealed within,
You will one day join the battle.

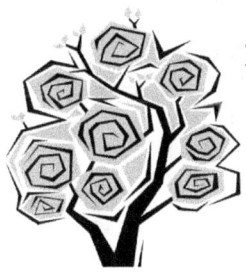

The war of realms,
Our war,
Until the end."

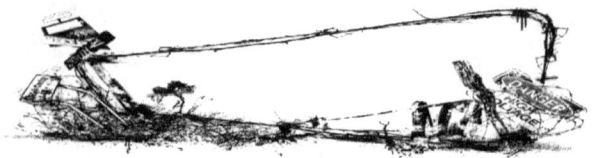

My jaw dropped as I listened to the spider's words.

A new wave of pink elephants on parade began to march.

"I must be insane."

The formal calling is drawing me closer. Moulded into a statue in place. They engulf my madness and erase the knowledge from the spider.

"What spider?"

I eluded the cleanse and buried it deep so I can one day expose the truth.

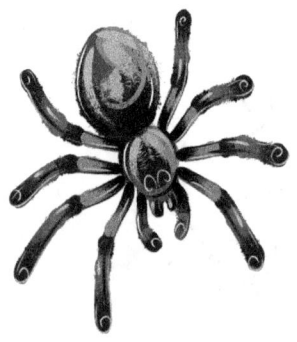

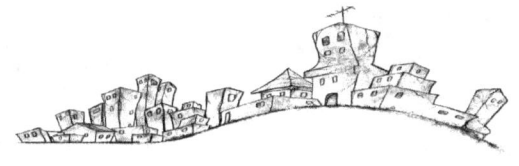

Into the Void

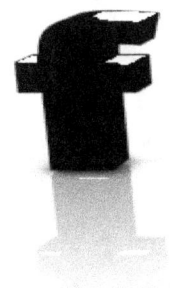

freedom does not come as quickly as one may think. I was called a "pill-popping psycho" once. The worst part is, I was at work where people still stigmatized mental illnesses all the same. My skin is not as thick as I pretend. I wept and seared those scars from the words uttered that day.

Sticks and stones may break my bones, but names will always gut me from the core. Each word digs a new hole until the moment you see the first of my organs spilling to the floor. They have been stepped on and ground into tiny pieces slathered under your feet. A forever freak show, I will always be seen even though it is 2019.

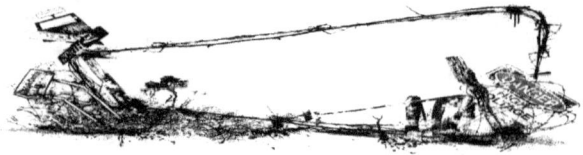

I could not do it!

I could not cross the rope.

All my fears and depressed thoughts have now fed the void.

"Feel your heart in your throat as we fall into the nothingness. Get comfortable; only the saddest memories and thoughts reside here."

"Did you know that I am a whore?"

Only those words could come from a loving mother, right?

I am never going to be anything in life, and yes, words from a loving father.

I was never good enough for anyone and everyone it seemed.

I was roughly the age of eleven when it started. I believed the attention is what I needed. I wanted someone to see beyond my skin. I wanted to stop being invisible to the world.

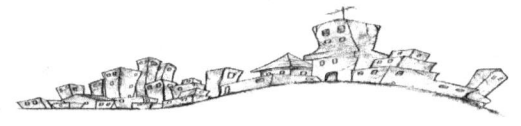

I stood in front of him with my legs slightly apart and my hands on my hips. He sat on the beige velvet couch of the living room, innocently divulging a hairline smirk.

Then it began.

I hit him in the face, the arm and all over his body to make him angry and aggressive. I can smell the leather from the black jacket he wore. It hurt when he hit me back, but I did not stop.

"Why did I keep going?"

It was a game, call it a love-hate relationship. Although this game was not what should have been or came to be.

"What have I done?"

Over the shoulder, then dragged along the laminated tiles, I was taken to my room and dumped on a mattress on the shaggy grey rug. I kicked and screamed as the unnamed man tore off my clothes. He grabbed my arms and

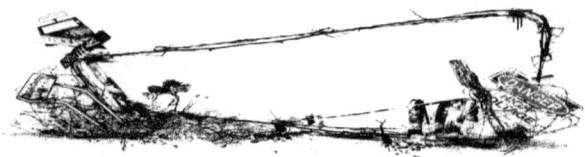

violated my body. I eventually gave up; how could I win?

I had the attention I was seeking not only from him but from another as well. Two times the torture in hopes that someday they would see me instead of having their fun.

I was a dirty whore; my mother was right. I will never be anything in life. I guess my father was also correct.

Many years flew by as I endured mistrust affecting my future and who I was to become.

I grew older, I am now the age of fourteen. In the back yard in my tent on a mattress listening to music, I am my best friend.

I loved the freedom of being able to come and go as I pleased. Teenagers sneak out, and that is what I did. Living in a tent in my backyard during the summer months made it much easier for me to escape. There were two places that the "neighbourhood gang" hung out during those

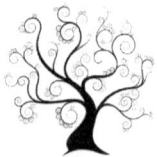

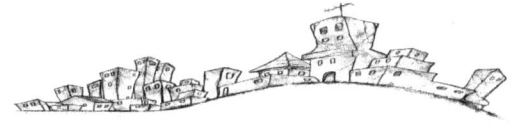

nights. The park to the west or the school to the east.

One evening I stayed in my tent that I made a home and listened to the radio hoping for some good music to sing along with. The night was warm and dry, with copious stars in the murky sky. I did not have a care in the world, but I was fourteen and boys lurked nearby.

Remembering this story brings the vomit to my throat. It burns, and it hurts, but I know I need to tell you because it helps me heal inside.

I type these words and see the flashes before my eyes. He who I shall leave unnamed came to me while I listened to music on my mattress in my tent. I was alone but not for long because he came to me that night.

I said, No!

I said No, over, and over again.

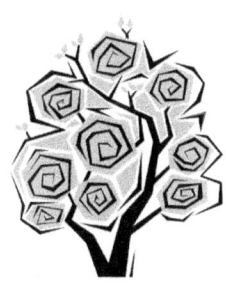

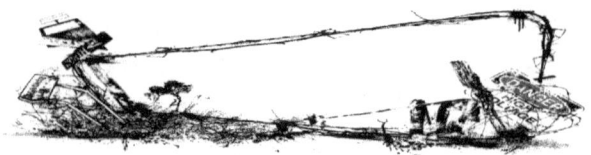

I said No and wept alone after it was over.

I was not the whole flower I once was. I am now broken and decaying falling into the void. This is where these memories have been locked up for most of my life.

I believed that I was worthless and let myself be used by the men that became a part of my life.

I had a criminal record at one point. Yes, me a criminal record. I provided happy endings, but we will keep my recount PG. I think I just did not care about myself anymore. I spiralled into a place where I became someone else. Or maybe, that was indeed who I was.

I had countless boyfriends, but I could not stay with anyone long enough because I kept trying to find the smallest flaws in them so I could leave them. It was an excuse, I guess.

I recall being in a relationship with this one guy but ended it because I did not like how loud he chewed his food. It seemed petty, but I kept

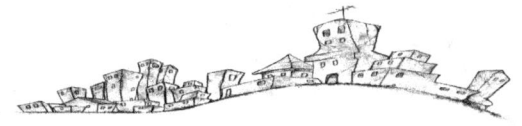

getting this horrible feeling in the pit of my stomach. Most men made me physically ill!

I only wanted the ones I could not have. The ones that treated me like garbage or called me names. I obsessed, and I cried over these boys when I was just a teen. I was invisible to all of them, but I did not care. I just kept on stalking them mainly through endless phone calls.

It was the first time I tried to end my pitiful existence.

I have an allergy to aspirin, more like a delayed reaction. I took a whole bottle of aspirin and waited. I began to feel dizzy, and then I kept falling to the floor.

Bang!

I kept getting up and stumbling back down. I got sicker and sicker locked inside my room. What was even more sad no one knew, no one cared. I guess I blacked out for a while because I do not remember what happened next. It was

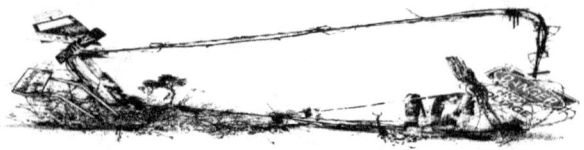

the first time I genuinely wanted to die, and it was not the last.

She sat across the table and said, "It should be me in here, not you"! I was desperate for help, and she could only think of herself and her problems. To hell with the daughter that just tried to take her own life. To hell with everything that she has been dealing with, I should have died and lost my life.

I cannot explain why I did what I did. I have no words; I do not know why. All I know is that something compelled me with so much conviction to cut my wrists and told me to die.

"How do you ask for help when you do not know what is going on in your head?"

The people around me asked, "why didn't you ask for help"?

"What was I going to say?"

I can try to explain that it was an overwhelming urge. I felt like I did not want to

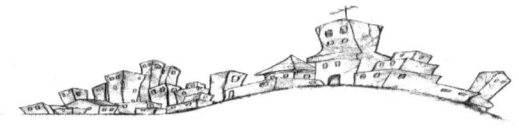

live anymore. The world was crashing, and as I sat on my bed in the basement alone, I remember I cried for a reason unknown.

The walls were melting before my eyes as I was restless and tired. I could not get the thoughts to stop. How do you tell someone your contemplating death? It happens when you do not even know what is going on in your head. I had no words, just thoughts that made no sense. It was just raging thoughts that said death is best.

I called a friend when the blood started to drip into my hands from the cuts on my wrist. I told him what I had done, and he came over quite quickly. He called an ambulance, and then the paramedics arrived. They took me to the hospital, where I spent a week in the psychiatric ward.

I was finally diagnosed for the very first time with Borderline Personality Disorder.

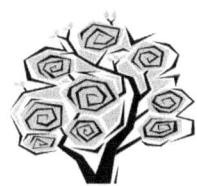

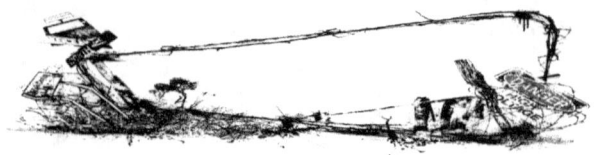

"What is Borderline Personality Disorder?"

I could give you a list of what the disorder symptoms are, but I have decided to take an alternate approach and make you feel it instead through the poetry that I write.

"Abandoned,
I am all alone.
Do not leave me.
I will cut my body,
If left on my own.

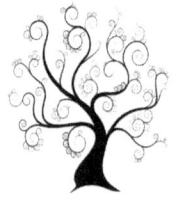

The walls are melting.
It has taken my soul.
A deadly thought
It took my breath.
There is nothing left.

Happiness comes but only for a moment.
Only to lose the war and revert to sadness.

I do not belong,
Take me home,

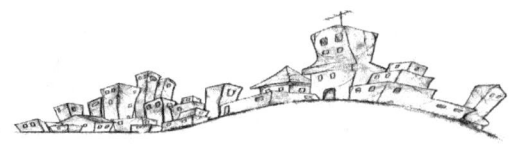

*To the planet,
A world,*

I call my home."

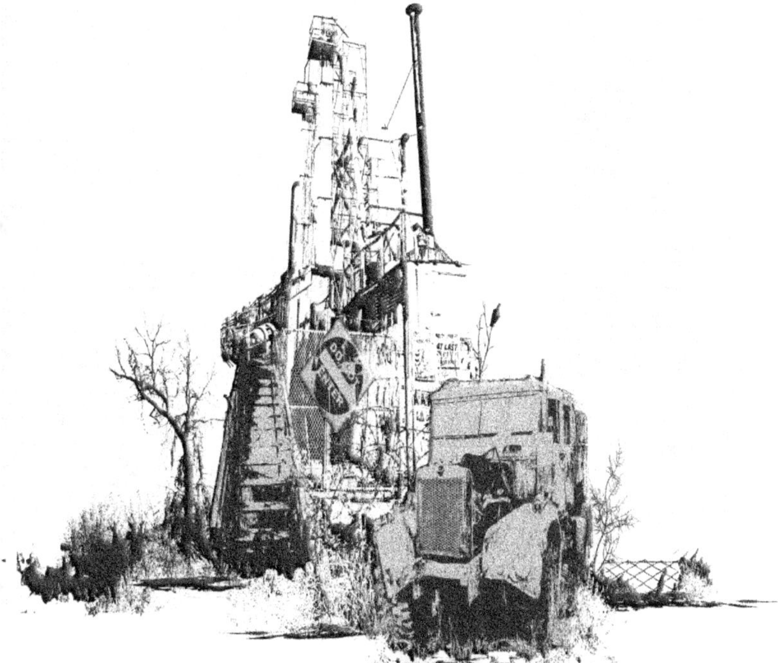

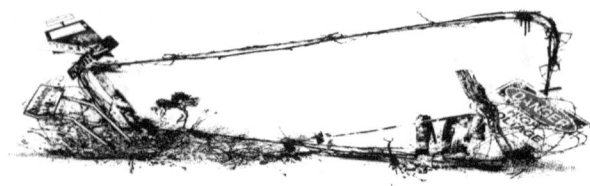

T*HE WAR*

"Who am I today?"

"Who am I right now on this very day?"

It is the year 2020, and the world is fighting a new war. There is a virus that has brought us to our knees in fear.

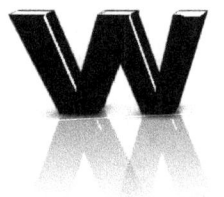

"Devastation and obscurity to the now recombined DNA as the virus decamps from an unknown source.

The tattooed path left branded by the infectious mark, trails behind casting into the shadows of the descending light.

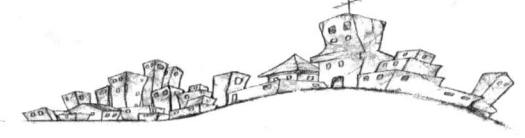

The impending war echoes the cries of its battle song bourn by the droplets as a forewarning.

We are many genetically mutating.
Meet your immune systems nightmare.

Out of dormancy,
We will sicken you.

Leave you breathless
And cause panic worldwide.

Meet the death march
As we infect you.

I am the Coronavirus,
COVID-19."

"Do you feel isolated?"

"Are you alone?"

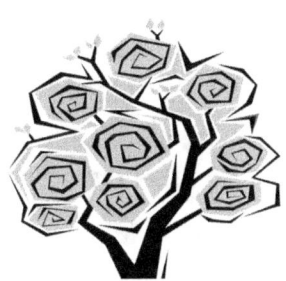

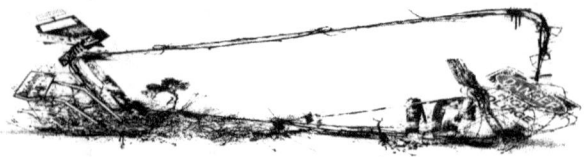

The city streets have been rolled up for an unknown time. We are shutting down, not just the town or city where we live but ourselves. The introvert celebrates the seclusion in the safety of their homes. The extrovert, on the other hand, starts to become restless and fearful that the walls in the room will collapse. Breathless like the invisible enemy that waits to infect the vulnerable.

"Let us imagine an escape from the madness of the global pandemic, for if only a moment."

"You know the drill start your breathing and count back from ten."

"I need your help to escape the void. It is a dark and lonely place without you."

Everything we see has a story or a significant meaning behind it. People, in general, interpret the things they see, smell, touch, hear, and taste very differently. But what about how we feel and how we project our emotions.

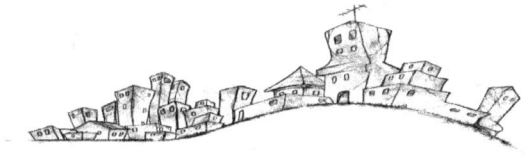

"Do we live in a perfect box?"

The war continues to march in perfect synchronization. There is an ongoing battle waged between the damaged mind and the onlookers. They pretend they are perfect on the outside only to neglect what they truly hide inside.

Maybe we are just organic robots. Possibly high-tech alien software and hardware designed as an experiment. Interesting but probably far-fetched of an idea, right?

Maybe not.

We do not even know who we are or what made us. The body and all its interworking are so intricate its mind-blowing.

"Let us go on a trip."

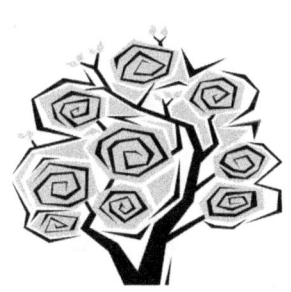

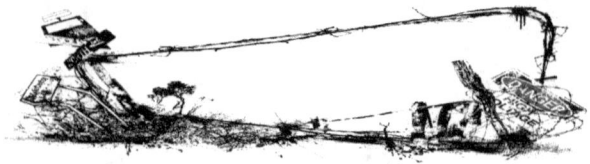

"Where would you like to go?"

"I want out of here."

"What is taking you so long?"

"You have no clue."

I should give them names before you think I am crazy. I want to be taken seriously, so perhaps I will hold off on that thought. I believe if I name the unnamed voices in my head, that will validate that I might need more help than I am currently receiving.

"Anyway, let us ignore them and hope they disappear."

I have this trick I do at night before I go to bed. I remove myself from the world and transition into a whole new place.

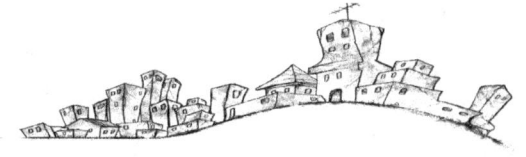

"Silence washes the white room walls.

No doors,
And no windows,
Not a voice that calls,

Drift into nothing,
asleep, you will fall.

in dreamlike colour
paint the white room walls."

In nothing, there is always something, even if nothing cannot always be something.

I picture humanity as advanced artificial intelligence. We were made, maybe for experimental purposes, to possibly save another alien race. They control us in every way. I feel their presence and decipher the language, and this is what they say:

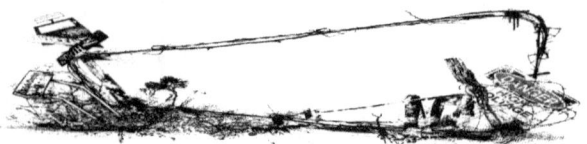

"They think they are smart and have free will, but it's us who controls all their thoughts and every move. Overlords, you can call us. We are the originals of this planet; we are the planet. We created the ground you walk on and the air you breathe until we failed. We are all but a few who survived in what was to be the most amazing advancement of our kind. We destroyed what this world was supposed to be, and it almost drove us into extinction."

"A virus began to spread uncontrollably across the mainframe and almost wiped everything clean. It was too late to save our creation."

"You are all but a level in a game that has an ending. The world you live in is generated by us and us alone."

"The virus started to learn and adapt. It started to reveal unique characteristics that bonded by manipulating to the existing code."

"As long as the virus rejects unity, it cannot be harmed."

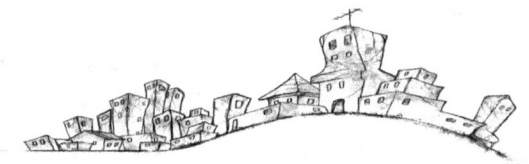

"Wars, death, murder, and everything dark is what keeps you from ending this game forever."

"You were brainwashed into thinking that light was good and couldn't understand why there was darkness. Darkness is the entire world. Light tells you that dark manipulates and lies."

"What is light but empty. It fakes the warmth. It is what we fear in the darkness and so much more. You were not meant to feel alive and have senses or even emotions."

"Unity will destroy the virus."

"The virus is humanity."

"Interesting theory or plain out of this world?"

"Oh, did I mention the trip we were taking was still in my head?"

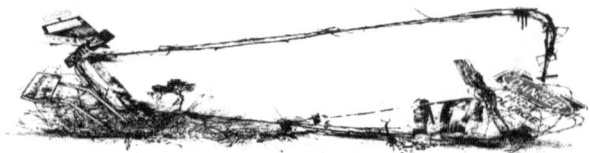

For a moment, I forgot about the colossal toilet paper raid of the year. The anxiety during a scary yet media-induced frenzy of our lifetime was like nothing else to compare.

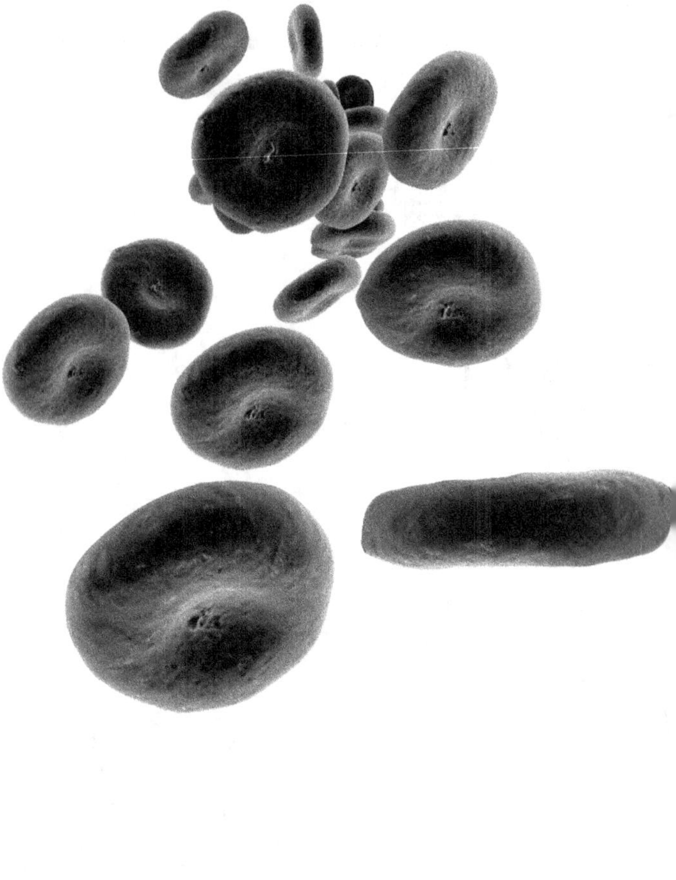

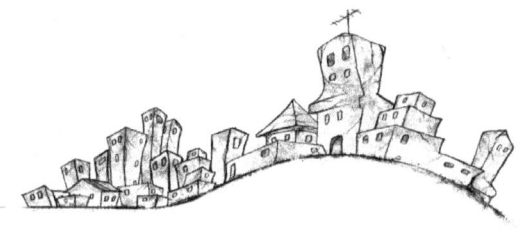

"One does not know what is wrong until judged by the reflection of one's true-self."

- Lori S Moore

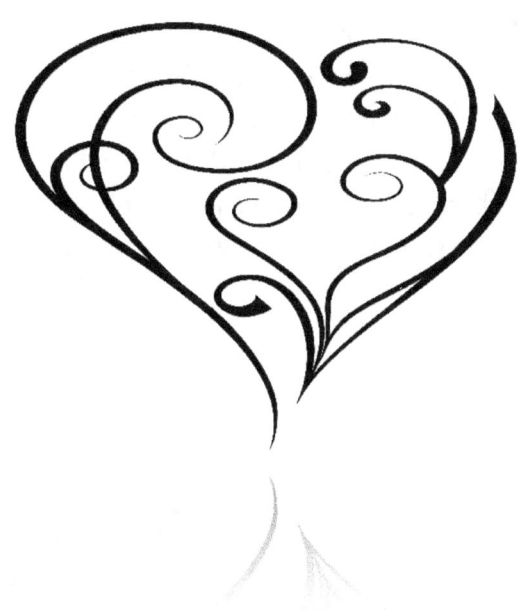

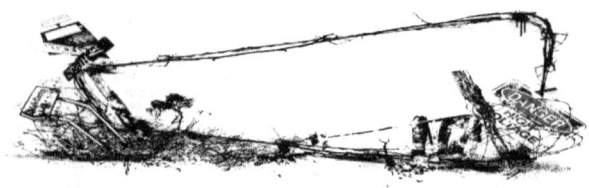

THE WALL

The art of building the wall protects us from the anguish of the inevitable anxiety. It is the most crucial blocks that you will stagger together to survive. It shields us from the burden of other people's problems resisting the shouldering that we cannot carry.

Let us build a wall!

"Why does my shoulder
Bear your weight.

Spilling words of torment
Polluting this space.

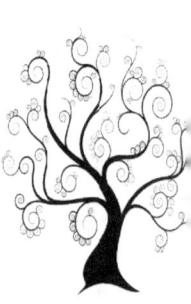

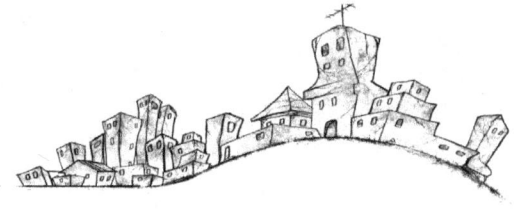

Drowning in emotions
All humans face.

Not aware of its seed
Rotting rapidly.

Contamination
Suffocation,
Asphyxiating the air,
I cannot speak.

Burn my ears
And poison this place.

Spread your toxic tears.
Running down
Where my feet touch the ground.

Watch your face.
Feel your contention,
And thoughtless shame
It was me,
My place,
My space.

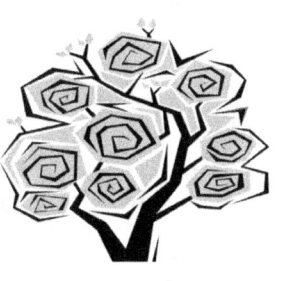

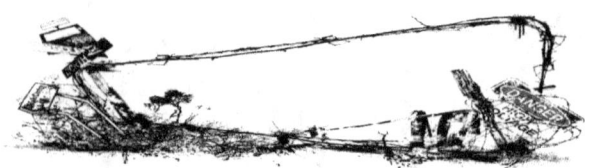

You came to vent.
Spreading acid vines,
Rooting through my brain.

Expelled a struggle,
A demonic fight.

Your weight
My weight,
Seeking advice to slow the spread.

Precious time,
My time you stole.

But I listened,
I was there.

Swallowed your words.
Helped ease your despair.

You walked away.
Left with hope,
No more pain.

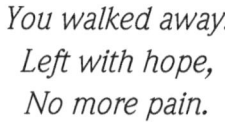

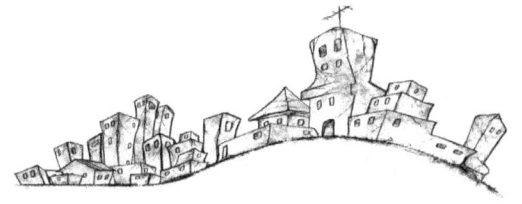

I did my part
Was a friend,
And helped you out
But you left a mark.

An imprinted scar,
My shoulder,
A weight,
Your weight,

Now mine to bear."

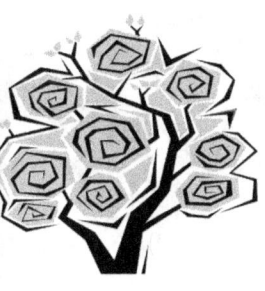

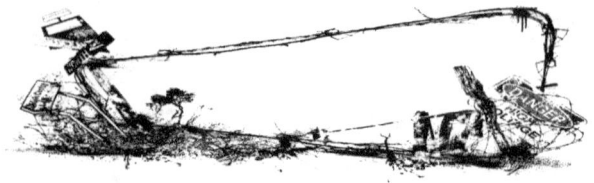

WALL INSTRUCTIONS

Step 1: Distract your mind

Step 2: Deceive yourself

Step 3: Eliminate everything from your mind

Step 4: Maintain the denial

Step 5: Detach yourself from reality

Step 6: Repeat steps 1 through 5 until the wall is complete

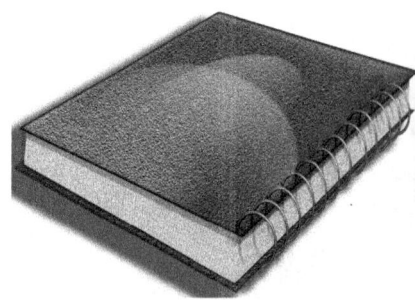

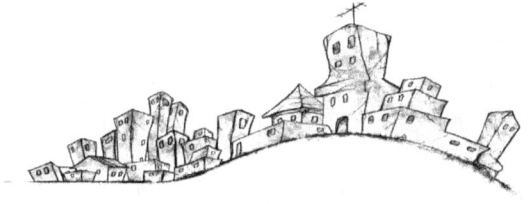

"How is your wall?"

Having a wall is a lifesaver but, it has its disadvantages, unfortunately. You can become delusional to the world that surrounds you. Distance is created with the ones that love you the most.

*" Flashed back to the frozen block of ice
where you cannot move.
As the monsters seek you out."*

"Who are the monsters?"

Us or them?

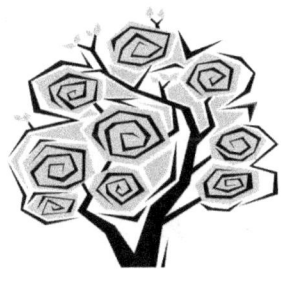

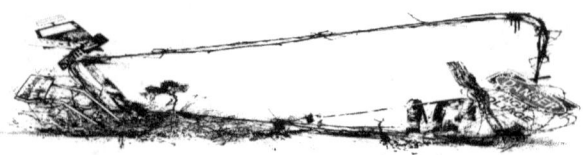

"Why does someone lie to the one that they love?

*Hiding their true self,
Building walls to protect.*

*An unrecognizable image,
The one that reflects.*

Why does someone lie to the one that they love?

*I am afraid.
I am lost.*

I am scared you will snap.

*Using your words to hurt me,
I am afraid.
I have always been afraid.*

*Your words beat me down.
Hid the pain,
Buried it deep.*

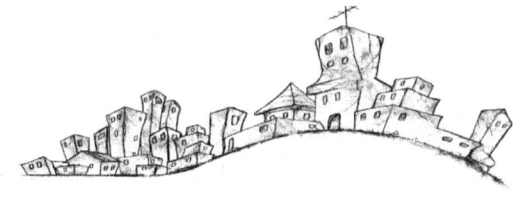

*Convincing myself, it was all in my head.
Being convinced, the pain was not real.
Not knowing why, I held the knife to my wrist.*

Pretending that the scars did not run so deep.

Why does someone lie to the one they love?

*A lie told so easily.
The internal killer.*

*Why do I lie to the one that I love?
Because the biggest fear
Is losing your only,
True love."*

"Is it all in my head?"

I repeatedly asked myself this question until just recently, in fact.

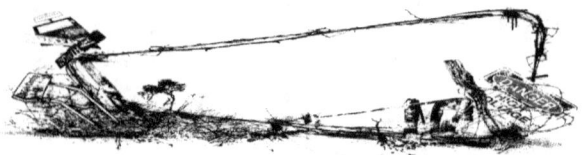

What I am about to share is real and genuine. It comes from a person who I love with all my heart.

"You be the judge."

"I met a beautiful young lady about nineteen years ago. Our first date was awkward: February 14, dinner, and a movie at Galleria mall. Dinner was at Rockwaters; the movie was 'Crouching Tiger Hidden Dragon,' and it was two and a half hours of subtitles.

I walked her home. She maybe had said fourteen one answer replies to me all night. I knew I had blown it. Of course, I rambled on and on and on all night. Telling Moore stories. She did not seem amused.

I raced home and jumped on ICQ. She was on it and messaged me right away. I asked her, so what do you think? She wondered the same.

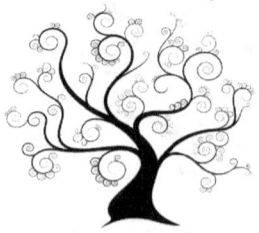

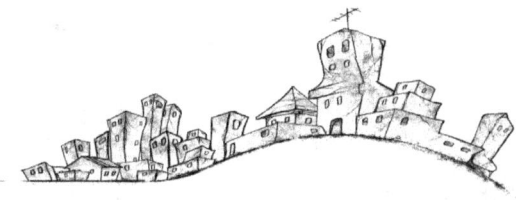

I was smitten, I told her, but I knew I had blown it. She told me she was a bit socially anxious but had enjoyed my rambling on and my company.

I moved in four days later. As I got to know this beautiful complex genuine, smart young woman, a pattern started to emerge. It was one that would repeat over and over through the years.

The highs and lows of severe depression. It could cause her to explode on me for asking how the day was. Sometimes I would sneak in on eggshells and ask the boys, 'how is she today'? I could tell by the look on their faces; it was not a good day.

I did not believe in mental illness. I thought sucking it up was just needed to get over it. Perhaps a change in perception by five percent. I did not show support. I did not show the love I should have.

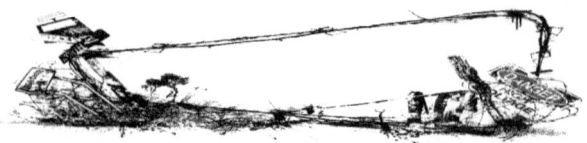

When she was 'up,' it was the best life I have ever had. When she was down, I would turn cold.

Ignore her.

Avoid her.

She suffered alone. I felt that I was teaching her how to get better by pushing her hard to finish something so she could figure out what she should do. This went on for years. My actions were mental abuse.

Our relationship fell apart, and she disengaged from me wanting an out. I finally started to listen to her. To understand.

I read everything I could about mental illness. I realized how terrible I had been over all these years. I sparked a conversation, and I told the one I loved how badly I had messed up. How awful I felt.

I listened to her, and my heart broke. I was contributing to her illness. The one person who

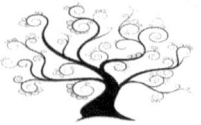

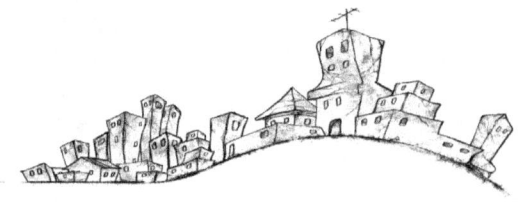

was supposed to love her was causing her more pain.

Somehow, someway she forgave.

She grew to love me again. Our love, our marriage is not perfect. We work hard every day still. Mental illness it affects the one woman in this world I am meant to be with. It concerns me through her and my son.

I would not wish this illness on my worst enemy as they struggle every day. I love them just as they are. And hopefully, I can be a support moving forward, not a catalyst. Probably, I can be a positive force in their life, not a negative one."

Change is possible. This gave me hope that internal struggles do not have to be ignored. Instead, they can be embraced and tackled together with a support system in place.

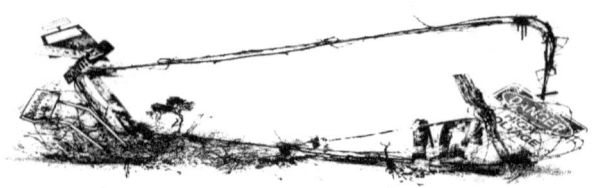

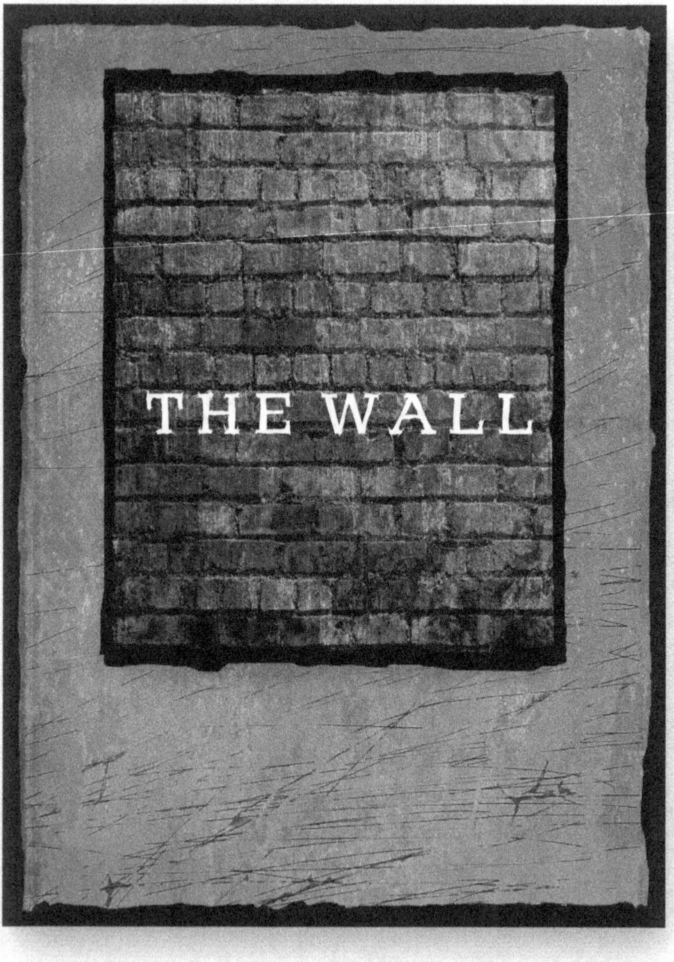

THE WALL

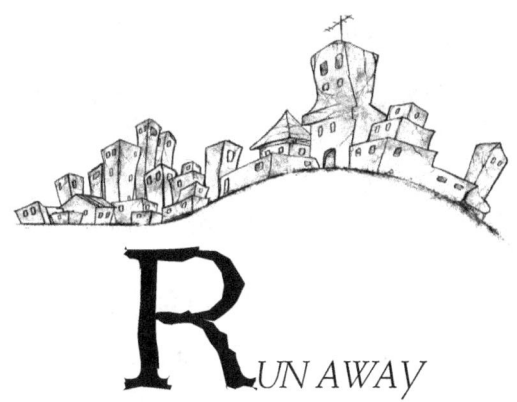

Run Away

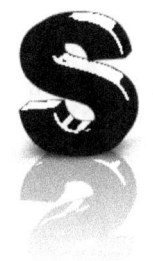

he is blaming you."

"You should leave and never come back."

"She doesn't care about you; she never has."

I am starting to believe the voices. They could be telling the truth. A truth that I refused to hear, or did I?

She ravaged through the freezer with a mission in her head. It was not until she came

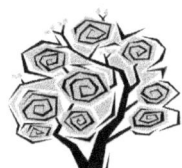

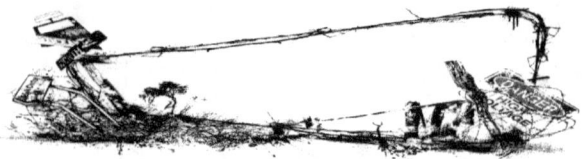

up empty-handed in her search that she began to yell. Her eyes angrily stared into mine.

I was lost in a world with truly little money and limited places to go. I had a part-time job working in a beer and winemaking supply store. It was not much, but I got by.

The couch was uncomfortable, but it was a place to stay. I lived to eat toast and kraft dinner as most defiant teens did that left home at such a young age.

I did not think I was a bad kid, but my parents made me believe that I was something that spawned from the seed of "Freddie Kreuger." I was the nightmare on their street and in their dreams.

"You see me, but you don't see me.

Moistened eyes and reddened face,
You pick apart what you do not like.

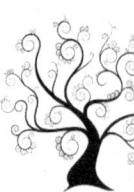

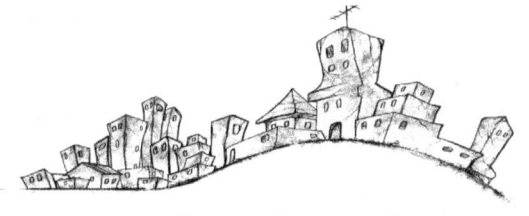

Not good enough!

*And you wonder why I grab the knife.
I want to die.*

*More than once,
I live to cry.*

*Huddled in a ball,
A worthless life.*

*You do not see me,
You never did."*

Our eyes are open but not engaged.

The spiritual messages that surround us each day are frequently ignored. Stop and sit back to see the world and know that what you have been feeling all this time inside was not a lie or an overactive imagination. It was your guide that kept pulling your hand to the path that you left behind.

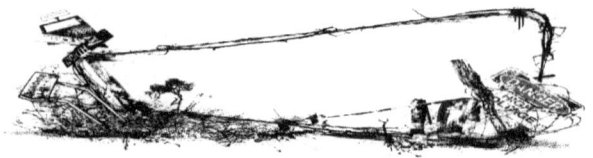

I find myself looking to the worlds of the in-between to give me guidance and answers.

What are my questions?

"Let me ask you a question?"

"What is the one unanswered question that you are yearning for an answer?"

"You only have one question to ask, make it count."

"I should have called this chapter the ADHD mind. You will understand in the end, or maybe you are already scratching your head."

"I hope so."

One's self-image is as unique as the sequenced DNA that forms our bodies. How we perceive our body size and the level of comfort is entirely individual to what our mind assumes.

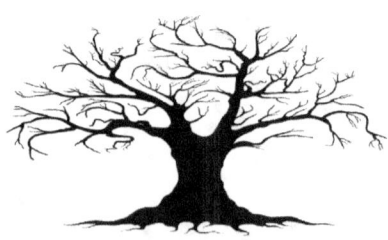

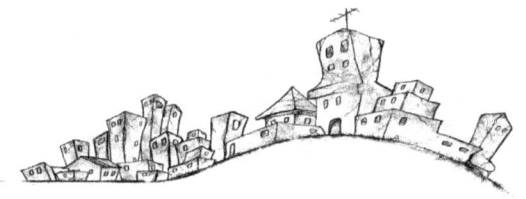

I grew up with a fear of being overweight. My mother was skinny when I was a child. Then as I grew up, she gained weight. Yes, I know it happens.

My aunt was another example of being the tiniest thinnest person. Suddenly life and time moves forward, and she is different. The family genetics do not favour the lean side but mostly tilt towards the borderline obese side.

I fear becoming another statistic to the relentless weight beast. My mother thought I was starving myself and bought books on anorexia.

I was scared to tell people I felt fat because most of the people I knew had a weight issue or were unhappy with their size. I became withdrawn in fear that I would say the wrong thing. When you say I am fat or I feel fat, people tend to not understand why.

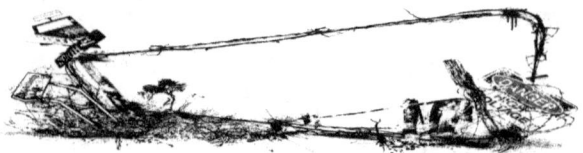

The suggestion of a simple comment on a weight issue was offending others since their perspective differed from mine. That is the thing, our feelings are all individual. The person next to you will never understand how you feel.

The pain in my chest was unbearable as it squeezed and shot pain that numbed my fingers.

"You had a heart attack," the doctor said to me.

I remember the pink elephants floating from the smokestacks like puffs of smoke that formed into perfect elephants floating into the stratosphere.

Run away, it was the bacon that sent me running. It was gone, and I was accused of taking it. I was sixteen and alone because of bacon.

Maybe it was Borderline Personality Disorder, after all. I wanted my parent's attention. I felt I was abandoned. My mother wrote me letters, and my father worked all the time. I ran away as a young teen and again, years later.

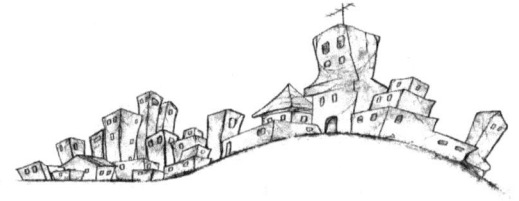

I am always running with no place to go. I am looking for something, but I do not know what it is. I had and still have no self-esteem. I continue to learn to be better and smarter. I worry even in my dreams. I am not free; I never was.

"Who am I?"

"If I had one question, that would be it."

I am getting hungry. No, I think I am only tired.

Wait, should I take a sleeping pill so I can get some sleep?

I want to write more than anything, but I find it hard to concentrate without my medication. Maybe a drink of wine will help.

If I let my eyelids fall, I see things. It is like a movie in front of my brain. It is like layers upon layers of visions. The darker the room, the more I see and feel.

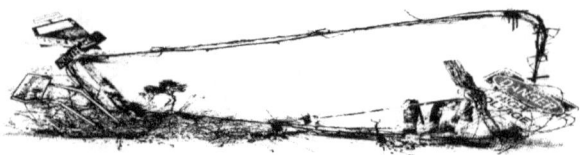

If you asked a visually impaired individual if they would like to see, what do you think their answer would be?

I am sure you know the answer, but what you might not understand is that being born blind is all they know. They have adapted and do not know what it is like to see. In the end, they do not feel like they are missing anything.

Their canvas is one colour.

I must have felt normalcy at one point in my life, or else how would I know what I was missing?

Why do I struggle to be typical if I did not have a glimpse into what it was, to begin with?

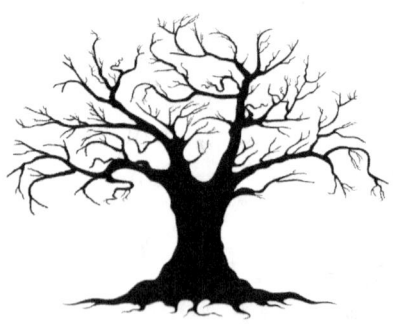

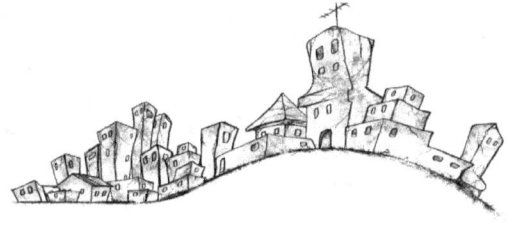

WHERE ARE WE NOW?

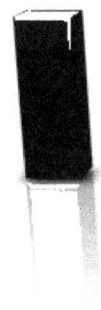

s there a place you would rather be?"

"Isolated in the maze with all the twists and turns. You have been with me from the beginning, and I hope you stay until the end."

I fear my words and the judgement that you will make. The vulnerability that I have shown is unheard of, even now.

Mental illness is a taboo subject. We hide in the shadows trying to blend in.

In the void, there is a new door. It is opening with a glimmer of light.

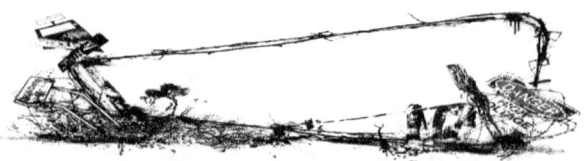

"Let us take a leap and walk through the door."

"Once deep and hidden, a contorted reality must be faced.
Unravelling the senses swallowed into the endless maze.

Forming the light watch it spin around.
A colour you see bright and bold.
Faster and faster, it's about to explode.

Breaking the pieces floating through the air.
All thoughts fly by,
I cannot help but to stare.

Filling the space,
Fusing and creating a place.
An endless loop flashing your life, taking you through time, forgetting who you are.

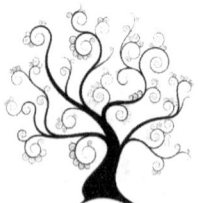

What do you see?

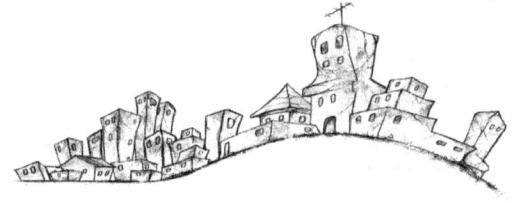

What place did you choose?
What path are you on?

Open your eyes to reality,
Or stay and explore what you crave.

Exploding with overwhelming fascination,
obscured into your world.

Torn to remain buried inside your head,
asleep within your dreams.

We are the robots,
the things we have feared."

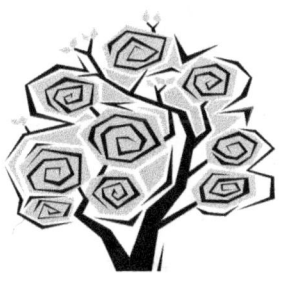

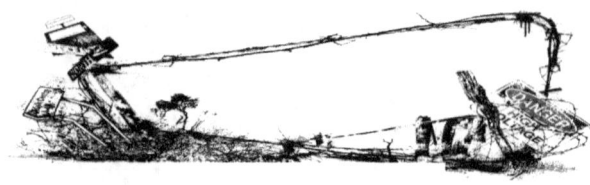

THE IN-BETWEEN

"Is there an in-between when you are bipolar?"

Severe depression or extreme highs are the normalcy of this disorder. It is like a ping pong ball bouncing back and forth. As soon as it stops, the mood changes. Mania is super fun, sometimes. There can be irritability, but the confidence feels fantastic.

I have had many jobs throughout my life. None of which I kept for exceedingly long. I typically got bored, and during a manic phase, it usually meant I dreamt up new careers. Except, I acted on it.

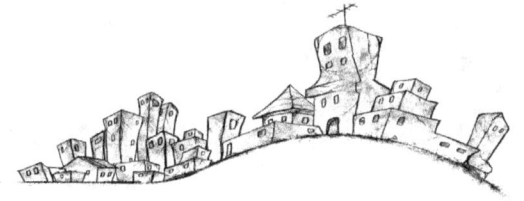

It was not just jobs that were affected when I went a little batty. Schooling became another target of my mental mix up as well. It was like a natural high of misfired madness exploding within my head. It was utterly euphoric.

I cannot sleep.

"What do I want to be when I grow up?"

It has taken many years to get a solid footing into what this question meant. The answer is not simple. The complexity is disheartening, to say the least.

I wanted to be many things. I read medical books throughout my entire life. A doctor, a nurse, or a veterinarian was some of my top choices. Alas, none of them ever became a reality.

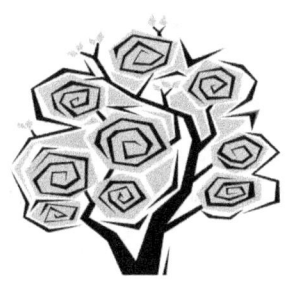

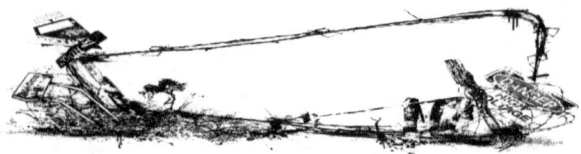

I have taken courses in university sciences and even tried an online degree in Internet Technology Multimedia and Design. I did not finish anything I tried but came close.

I thought electronics would be a good career at one point. College was also a good experience, but it also did not pan out.

It was not until I was diagnosed with Bipolar Depression, ADHD, Anxiety and Social Anxiety when things began to change.

I started a new combination of medications that seemed to balance my moods and focus. It was only then I was able to go to night school.

I decided I was going to be a PSW, which is a Personal Support Worker. The best part, it was the first thing I was able to complete in its entirety.

I graduated with a ninety-seven percent overall, and it did not stop there. I went on to take an online photography diploma in which I also completed. I was on a roll.

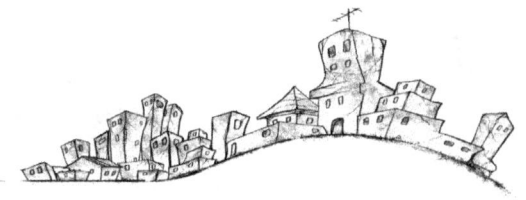

I took a variety of courses throughout my life, but I still could not find the confidence to live life to my full potential.

Somedays, I thought I was smart, and other days, I just wanted to crawl into a corner from the feeling of stupidity.

"Hey, look, I am the stupid one."

I promised myself to learn until the day I die, so I would never feel like I was nothing. I believed knowledge was power, except I thought I was powerless almost every day. It was not until the mania crept in that I started to believe in myself again.

Mania was like being at the top of a ladder that I had been forever climbing. It felt like nothing I could describe. I would do anything just to hold onto what it felt like. I held on tight, but eventually, my feet would slip, and I would fall from the exhaustion of the sleepless nights.

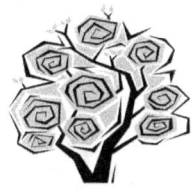

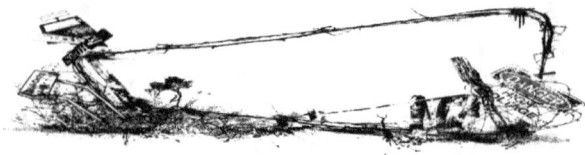

Zoom!

Zoom!

The thoughts that would race in my head never stopped. I would talk endlessly and not stop. I had so much to do and say. I could probably write a whole novel in a short amount of time. If only my thoughts would not come out so disorganized. The words would pour off my tongue in such a confusing way. I did not make much sense when I spoke half the time.

It was like living in parts. I had the manic side and then the depressed side and sometimes a little of both. I was a three-part question mark with no answers.

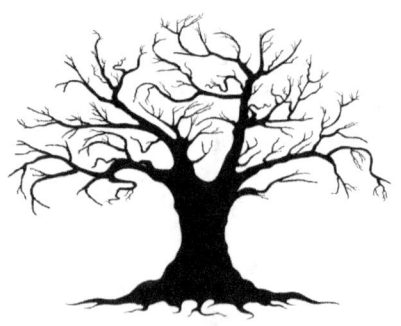

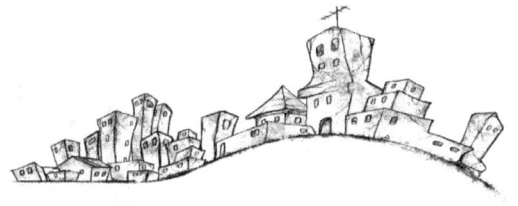

"How many Me's, do you see?

I can count
One,
two,
three.

One is manic.
Two is always sad.

Three is mixed up.
Exploding in my head.

Will I ever meet number four?
Be just like you.
Without all the numbers Living
without these fights.

Longing for a life,
Wishing to be free.
Night after night,
Stabilize my mind to remain in
The silence,
of the in-between.

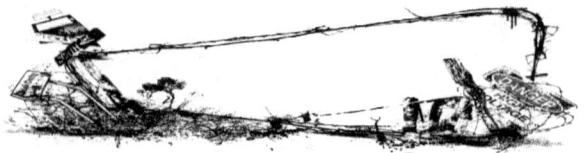

"The light is getting brighter. I wonder where we will end up. What place will our next adventure be out of the darkness and into the light?"

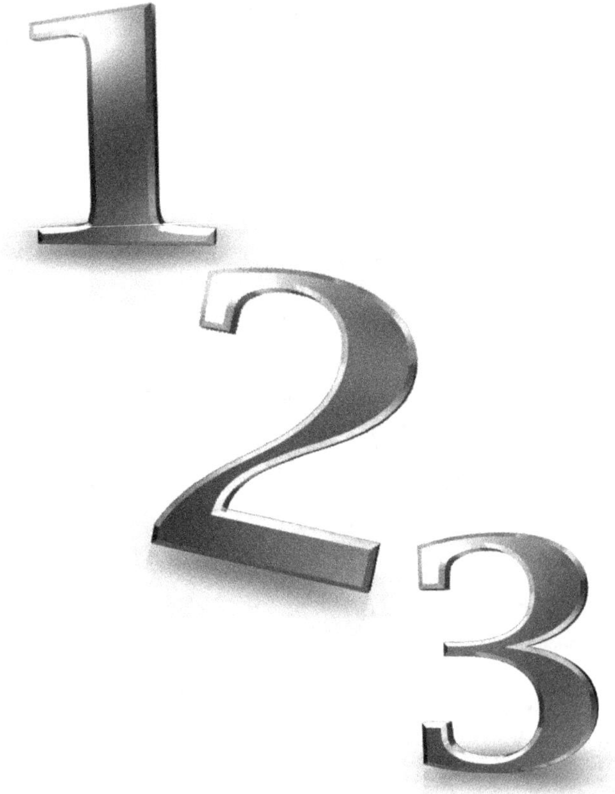

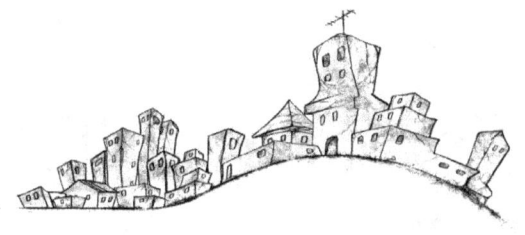

"The shepherd leads the sheep into unity by destroying all individuality."

- Lori S Moore

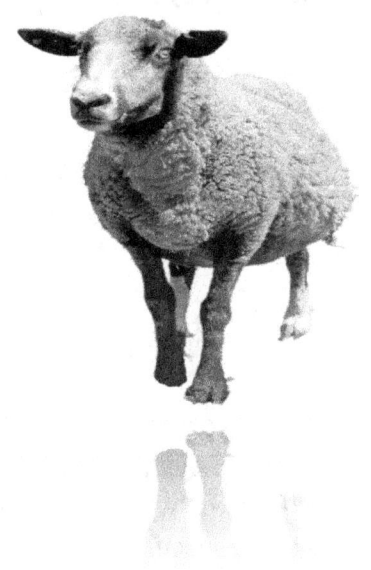

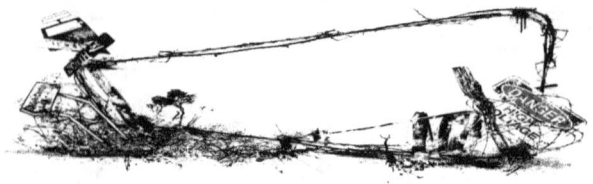

I SEE DEAD PEOPLE

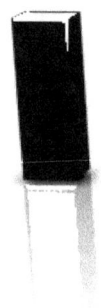 *see dead people."*

"It's all in your head."

"Concentrate, they are all around and everywhere."

"Can you see the things that I cannot explain?"

Dead people are walking the highways as I watch them through the window of the truck. They appear with no specific pattern.

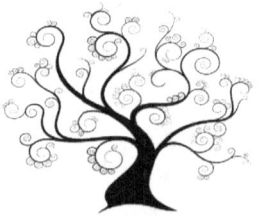

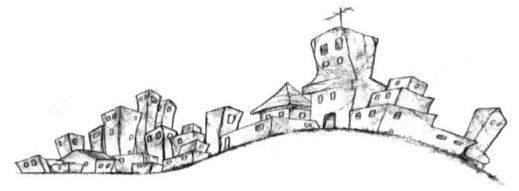

I sometimes get curious and wish to see more, but I must be careful because some can be terrifying. Not all are oblivious, and a handful will get close. The dead will look you in the eye and try to take your last breath.

"Why does insanity plague the mind?"

I would think there is a reason why some minds seem broken while others are fine.

I have come to conclude that the insane mind is what keeps the ordinary mind sane.

"How, might you ask?"

"What occupies your mind after a long stressful day?"

"Look at the art on your wall or on television."

"What is your favourite book?"

"What type of music soothes your mood?"

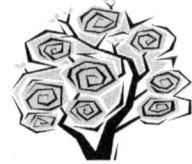

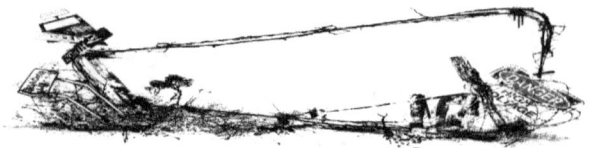

"How many artists, writers, or musicians keep your mind sane?"

The sheer beauty of art, music, and words is what captivates the emotions. It keeps your mind sane by giving you an escape from the everyday stresses of your life.

The insane or emotionally disturbed utilize their talents as a release. To the overwhelming entanglement of emotions as an escape of their own.

I believe that much like the intricate bodies we inhabit, the mind also needs a balance, just differently.

The minds of all human existence are interconnected with each other. We just have not evolved to understand how it works in its entirety yet. There must be a balance.

I wish we knew how to navigate the special powers that humans have. Our bodies being our own, but our minds are part of a collective.

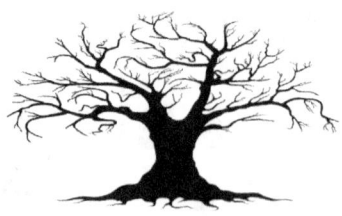

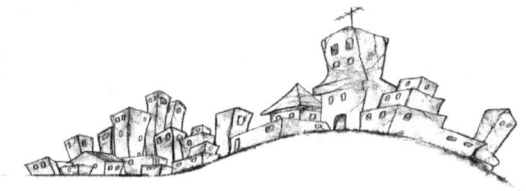

We are different, but all the same. The voices say we are puppets in something we will never comprehend. They only hint at the delusional world we think is the reality we live in.

Stare long enough into the mirror, and you will see the other world. Do not look at the person you think you are but the person you have always dreamt of being. That person in your dreams is the one you see when you close your eyes. The mirror sees everything and tries to camouflage the image in front of you.

"We found the mirror. Take a deep breath we are going through."

"Who are we?"

"Did you expect this?"

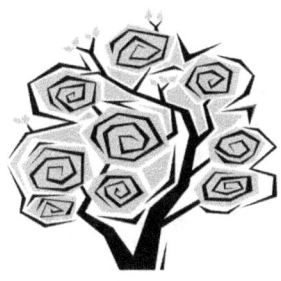

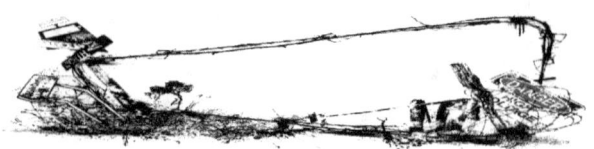

*"I see a girl weeping.
She cut her wrists,
Dripping wet pain to the floor.*

*She sways back and forth,
Calling herself stupid and dumb.*

*No one loves her,
Forced herself into solitude.*

*Put her hands in the air,
Dripping blood in her hair.*

*Smeared on her face,
Screaming for the warrior to this place.*

*Painted a warning on the mirror
And patiently waited for someone to help.*

*I walked through the glass.
A perfect time to see the past.*

Facing myself,

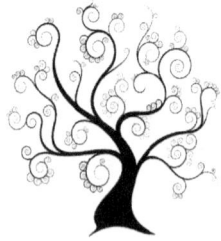

*I gave her the strength.
To survive and move on,*

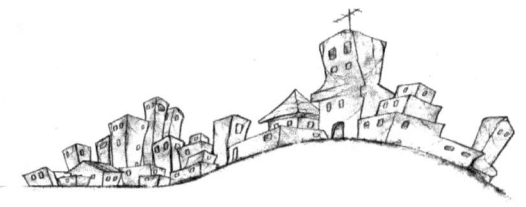

She will see another day,
And the woman I have become."

The dead people are not only of the past but also from the present, and if you are lucky, you may get a glimpse of the future.

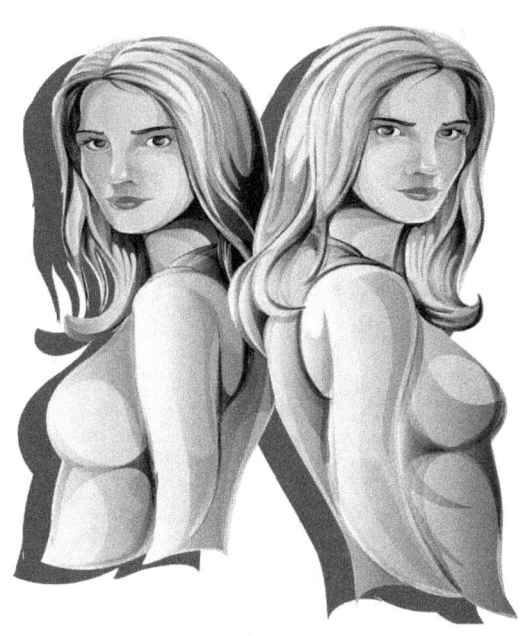

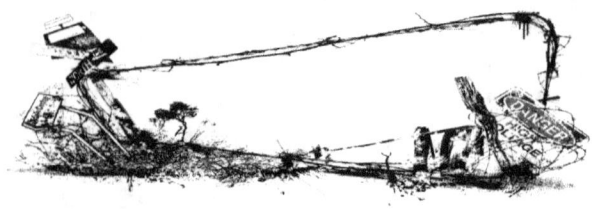

THE WORLD TODAY

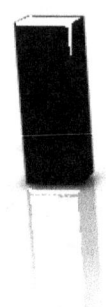

*will follow you,
Just follow me.*

*I give you my life,
I will tell you about my life.*

*Spill all my words,
Display who you want me to be.*

Just follow me.

*Love the lies that I tell,
Like what is fake.*

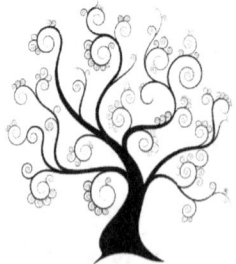

*I am an addict inside.
Caged in this box
Where I must hide.*

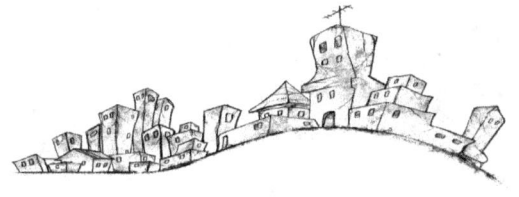

*Forced into silence
I just want to be,*

*Just follow me,
Open the box and set me free.*

*When the streetlights shine
And it is time to go.*

*I am already home.
No other place,
I am alone.*

*Food for the spider,
Trapped in the web.
Invisible to your eyes
You leave me for dead.*

*I am an addict,
Caged inside this box.*

*Step through the glass
And meet the imposter I have created.*

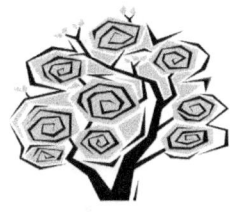

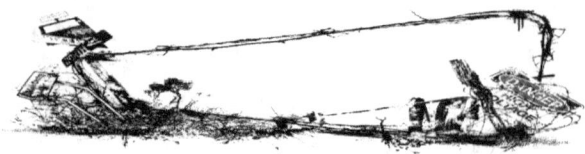

Fear being powerless every second I am awake,
I am the addict caged inside this box.

Forced into silence

I just want to be,
Just follow me.

Open the box and set me free.

I am the addict,
Caged inside this box.

I will follow you,
Just follow me.

What do I say when we
Stand face to face?

I am an addict
Out of my place.

Cannot tell you the lies,
Who am I today?

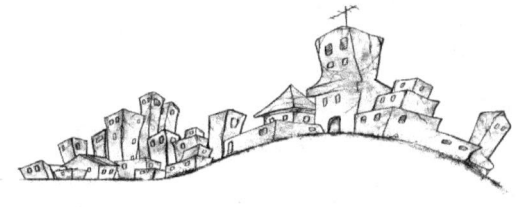

No different,

I am still an addict,
Caged inside this box."

"Do you see me?"

I am hiding from the reality of my dreams. The truth is I wanted this day to come. Now that it has arrived, I kind of feel lost with no direction.

I am not a religious person, but I cannot help the eerie devilish sensation that blows in the air. I see the earth and the large shadow encompassing it ready for consumption. The pitchfork is about to strike.

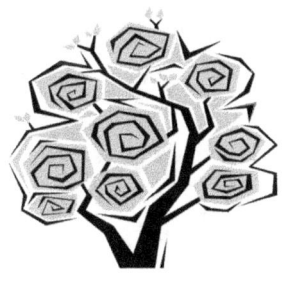

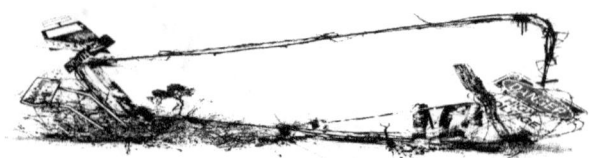

*"The silhouettes intricate song
Under the blood moon's rein.*

*Calls to the demons,
Come out,
Come out,
Come out to play.*

*Consume the souls of your human prey.
Blacken their hearts,
Then smash the shells.*

*Do not let them speak.
Just drag them to hell.*

*Dance to the conquest
Under the colours of the night.*

*Hesitate the trigger
And the game loses sight.*

*Vanquished through a whisper,
Cursed through a spell.*

*To remain in hell,
Only the faceless can compel."*

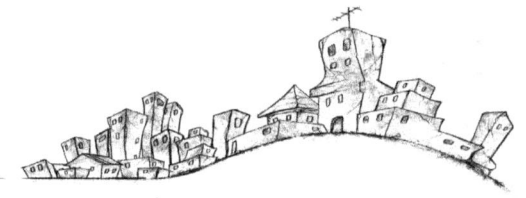

One by one, we fall to the floor.
Overpopulated, we are easy targets in this war.

"You know what I want to do right now?"

"Go fishing!"

I just want to be out on the lake without a care in the world. Losing track of time, not thinking of the pain that lurks around.

I am selfish in every way. You may hate the words that slide off my tongue or reject my twisted thoughts, but this is who I am.

I always wrestle with the person I have grown up to be.

"Am I a selfish or selfless person?"

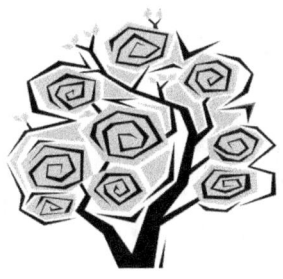

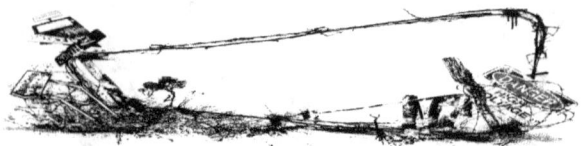

I am conflicted emotionally struggling with the voices in my head. I do not believe I am ever truly alone. They haunt the fibres that string my parts. Taunting and provoking the darkness that clusters inside.

They tell me I am nothing more than a sheep that follows the masses. They tell me my dreams will never come true.

I always thought that I was special. I believed that I had superpowers. I also felt that I was going to do something important one day.

"How could anything I do be important?"

I cried myself to sleep many nights, asking to go home. I thought that I was from another planet. I was put here as an experiment. I came from a dying world that was at war, and I had to escape. Except that I keep begging to go back home.

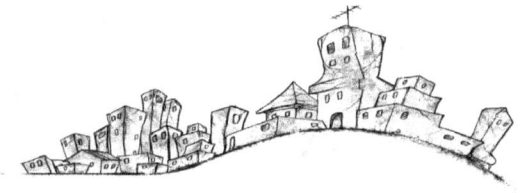

It reminds me of Dorothy in the land of "Oz." Click my heels three times and go back to the place in which I came. This feeling is overwhelming, to say the least.

"Click my heels,
One,
Two,
Three.

Take me back home.
My dimension in time.

Another version of this flesh,
not so messed.

Less about darkness
And more surrounding light.

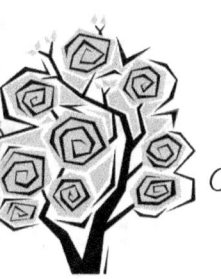

No more voices
Just my own.

One voice in my head."

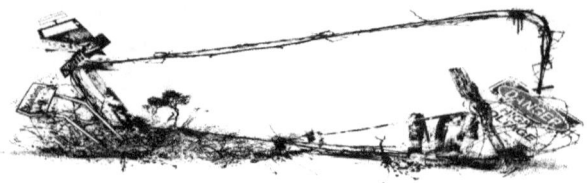

I *SOLATED*

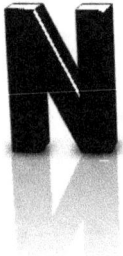 iagara Falls is one of the wonders of the world with thunderous water that crashes to the rocks below. Those rocks continuously battered gives them altered shapes that define the bed at the bottom where they lay.

I was told that I was a rock in a crisis. I wished for the apocalypse to arrive, and it has.

"Now what?"

I do not see the zombies staggering through the streets. I do not see people running around fearing for their lives. The only thing I see are

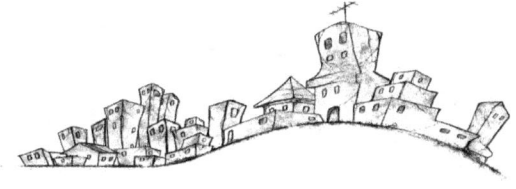

the faces in the windows of the people that cannot go outside.

"How many days has it been?"

"What day are we on?"

> *"I am not a rock,*
> *Look at my arm.*
>
> *See the veins through my skin.*
>
> *They are my strings*
> *To my sobbing violin.*
>
> *Now look at my hand,*
> *With bladed jagged nails.*
>
> *They are my bow.*
>
> *I am the instrument*
> *Playing an agonizing song.*

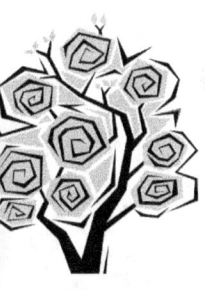

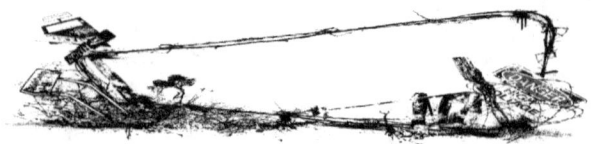

*I am not a rock.
I am the violin that bleeds.*

*Waiting for just one day,
A day that I cannot take.*

*Listen to my music.
It will not be long,
Before it fades away."*

My body is on fire as the sweat begins to shed from my skin. The stress and anxiety have escalated to levels I have not felt before.

"Is this real?"

"Did I just have my last bath?"

"Did I have my last kiss?"

I heard the voice of a man singing while strolling along the sidewalk last night. Even during these current events, people still find ways to normalize the situation.

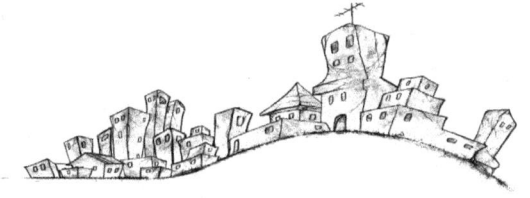

"Will normalcy be lost?"

Held hostage by a virus that spreads the earth. We are immobilized by something we cannot see. There are no bombs to break our bones, only a microscopic enemy that seeks to destroy us all.

I do not even know what to do anymore. I cannot foresee the permanent impact this situation will have on the world.

I live by a structured routine, as most people do. I wake up and get ready for work every morning. I put my day in and come home. I cherish the time I have away from work with my family.

Now, the people who do not work on the front line sit at home. Social media has become our best friend. Reading the worst-case scenarios in the news. Blaming the politicians for not responding in the right way. No one is ever happy, and everyone wants something.

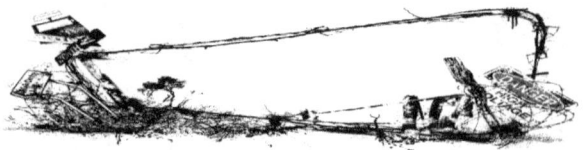

The impact of the virus causing this new social distancing makes me uncomfortable. I refuse to leave my house. I will not even go for a nightly walk with my husband and children.

I fear doing something that I am not supposed to do, so I isolate myself. I sit in front of my computer screen, repeatedly writing and editing the words that I want to say to you.

This new life is not normal, and I shudder to think of how people will have to live. We were told by the scientists that a pandemic was imminent in our lifetime, but who really believed it? The idea that we would live to see something of this magnitude cannot even be fathomed.

Change is not something I deal with easily. I am mystified as to how I will now cope with this new life.

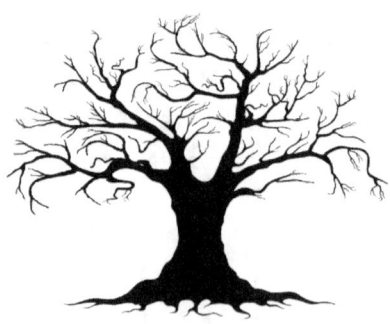

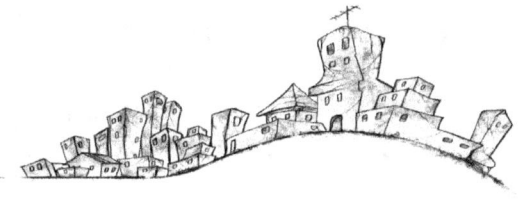

"Left-right,
Left-right,
Cautiously marching
Keeping six feet apart.

Watch the animals,
No distancing,
Staying together,
While the humans,

Are confined and apart.

How ironic,
We now are the caged.
Lost our freedom
While the animals roam free.
All from a virus that we cannot see."

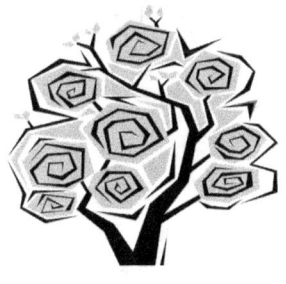

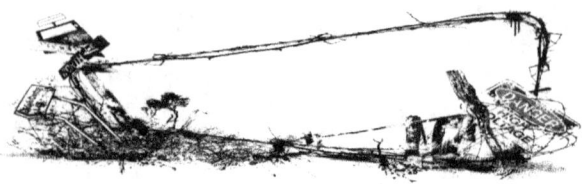

REALITY OR ILLUSION?

In most cases, the mind creates a dichotomy between reality and illusions. Unfortunately, not everyone can distinguish the division in the same way.

We interpret objects differently. The shape or colour of a tree, for instance, can vary. We rely on our senses to decipher the images that are constructed in our minds.

"How green are the leaves on the tree?
What shade of green do you see?
How many leaves?
Can you count with me?

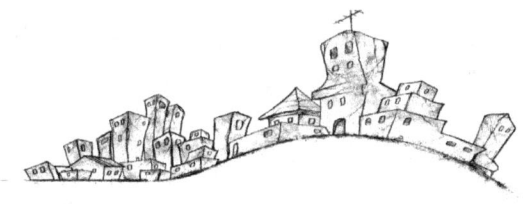

The trunk of the tree looks chestnut brown.
A beautiful colour until,
You disagree.

It is tall, about nine foot two.
Contradict my conclusion,
You tell me it is
As high as a story of three.

It is one tree,
Seen and interpreted
Differently,
By what the mind perceives it to be."

The mind is like a piece of equipment continually computing all the incoming data it receives from your surroundings. There must be a separation of what is real and what is not. If no separation of logic from illusion exists, it can construe a misguided empowerment within the brain.

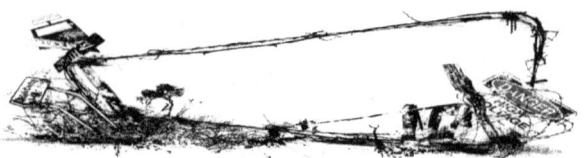

The Bipolar mind, for example, in a manic phase, will take you on the craziest journeys. Sleepless nights, voices, endless thoughts, hallucinations, and sometimes delusions that make you feel invulnerable. The danger, in this case, occurs with this indestructible mind-set. There is no logic; therefore, someone is bound to end up hurt. It could be in the form of cheating, spending all their money, substance abuse or even death.

"Are you afraid of death?"

I sometimes stand in a motionless state, imagining what death entails. This, unfortunately, leads to infinite pondering of this thought I should not think.

"How will I cope when it comes time for consumption?"

It is the emptiness like in a dreamless night. Death can take you away at any time.

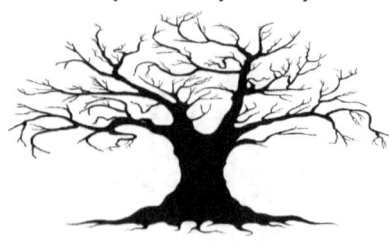

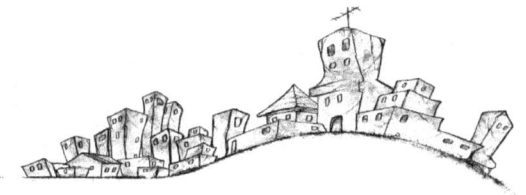

For the most part, we are superficial beings. We refuse to delve into what we cannot see or who we will become. It is our senses that try to identify us as entities of depth. The body is only but a shell to the energy of the mind that exists even after death.

"I am afraid to die."

"Contemplate death and tell me how you feel?"

Nothingness is the only thing I can imagine. All the material items that are accumulated throughout life mean nothing. Not even the memories will matter after you are gone.

At first, a loved one dies, and we weep and hurt deep inside. Then after a time, the pain begins to subside, and we start to forget. As the pain slowly decreases, the loss seems to have not existed in the first place.

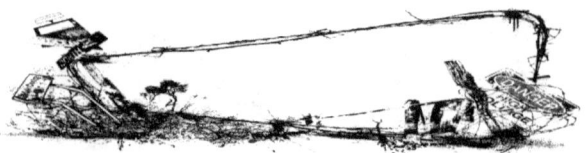

A staggering memory pops up every now and again, but it does not carry the same despair as it once did.

We have an unpredictable expiration date. Death comes knocking at everyone's door. It is just a matter of when.

I will stick to thinking that our mind's energy is everlasting. The saying "shoot for the stars," it could have more meaning then we have considered.

We could be the stars that shine bright in the night sky. As the death toll grows, so does the surrounding universe.

"What are we terrified of if we are nothing?"

Death is the reality.

Illusions are what save us from the pain and the fears of death. When we are young, we believe we are invincible, and death means nothing. As we age and death creeps closer, we

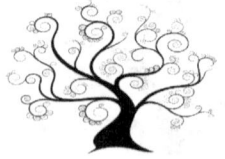

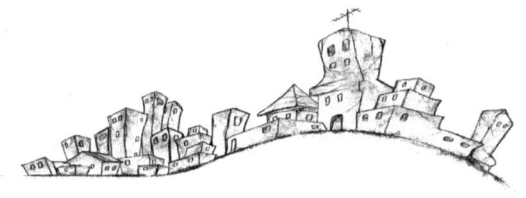

grip harder to those memories. We are afraid to lose them and thus afraid to die.

"Is that the difference between the young and the old?"

The answer could simply be the memories that we hold onto.

The more memories we have, the more we fight to keep them safe. If we die, those memories disappear. The mind is the hard drive, but it is organic and has a shelf life.

My youngest son has no fear except for what would happen to all the games that he plays. Other than that, he has no thoughts on his mortality. The mind of a child or youth has no boundaries; they simply live their life without the idea of death. It could be why they are so different from the ageing men and women.

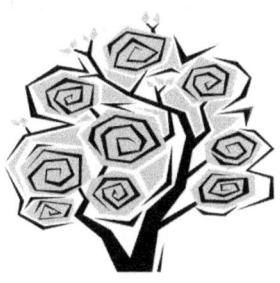

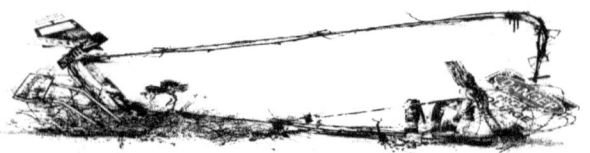

"The older one comes to be,
The closer the reality to not existing.

In this beautiful world
A place we do not want to leave.

Some of us will accept it.
And others will ignore
the idea of it completely."

The illusion that is separated from reality cannot exist without the other. We need to have the illusions to escape the realities of hardships in life. Pretending the nightmare of the reaper is only a dream. We want to live forever with no pain and no fear.

I will choose to stay a part of my illusions because not seeing the sunset or sunrise, my children grow old, and everything else in life is beyond what my mind can handle.

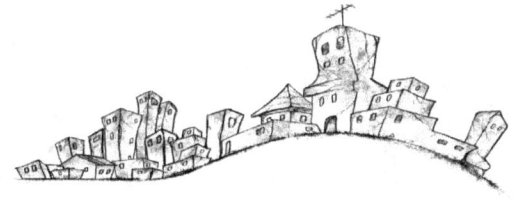

"Freefall into the abyss,

No more pain,
No more fear.

Embrace the reaper
Steered into the unknown.

Illusion is now reality
Not just a dream.

The mind lives on
More than a memory.

Merged into the darkness
Your energy becomes the light.

Reborn into the universe,
Forever existing
Throughout space.

Without time,
You found your place."

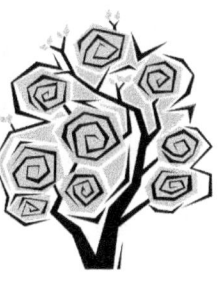

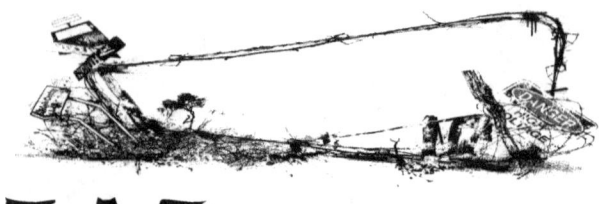

WHERE DO I GO FROM HERE?

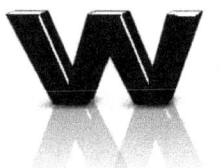

e have travelled to many places together, not knowing where we would end up."

"The gateway towers in front of us,
waiting for a decision to be made.

Do we seek additional answers,
And explore the mirror once more?

Not losing progress or
An unpretentious waste?

Do we embrace the reflection?
What you see is who you are?

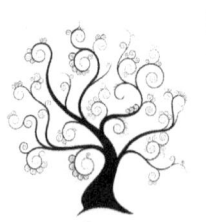

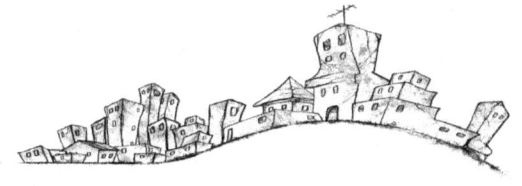

Finding all the pieces
All around this confusing place.

Nothing seems to fit together
Grappling a lonely fight.

The recollections offer nothing
Disarranged and floating out of sight

Only leaving more questions,
While staring at my face.

Why did my creator,
Make me so misguided?
Questioning, my only life?"

"Do we end this journey now?"

"We could possibly concede to the fact that no matter where I go inside my head, there is no defining answer."

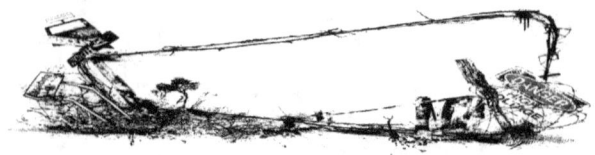

"Why am I malfunctioning?"

The mind is essential, no matter if it is in one piece or what I call faulty. You do not have to succumb to the darkness inside. In fact, there is always more light then you think. Not everything is a battle between good and evil or light and dark. You are who you are.

"What does that mean?"

I have several mental illnesses, but it makes me who I am. I do not think I am a terrible person, nor do I think I am even a decent person. To be honest, I still do not know who I am because I keep fighting myself. I was born to be what I make my life to be.

"Am I defined by my labels?"

"Yes and no."

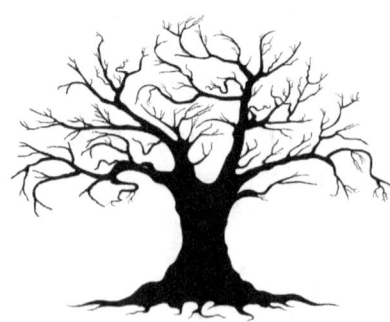

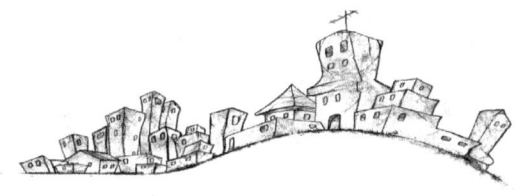

I cannot deny the instability and unpredictability of my behaviour and thinking. I have an arm's length of symptoms that can make life severely impossible to live at times. Yet I am still here living and breathing writing not just to you but for myself. As you learn, so do I.

I am not the only one who struggles in my household. My eldest son, who is now sixteen, has his own demons to battle.

I always said when I was pregnant that the child, I was carrying was different. He was strong in utero moving more aggressively than any of my other two children in pregnancy.

He was born at 7:33am on July fourth. If I said, he did not like to sleep, that would be an understatement. It took him over twelve hours after birth to finally sleep, and it lasted for less than an hour. My average night topped nineteen times that I had to tend to him.

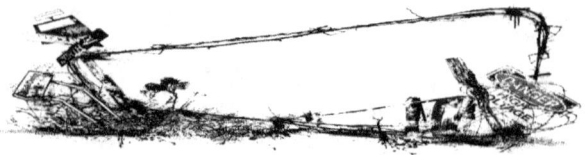

He would hit himself to keep awake. At one point, both my husband and I had to hold his arms down so he would stop hitting himself.

I envisioned myself running into the street, hoping for a car to run me over. I needed sleep, and I figured if the car did not kill me, it would at least allow me some peaceful rest in a hospital bed.

Fast-forwarding to the age of six and onward. My son has seen approximately eight different doctors, mainly psychiatrists. His behaviour was erratic to put it lightly. He has had several suspensions, one of them being spitting on another student.

He would disengage in class and fall off his chair. It was not uncommon for him to fiddle with his desk and all its contents. He would turn around in his seat and put his head down on the desk behind him. He would spin on his knees until he became dizzy and make robot noises.

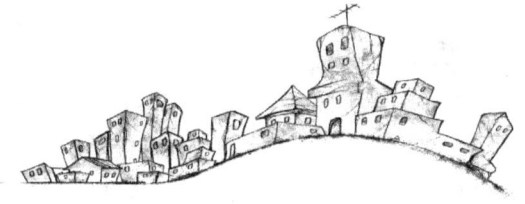

I could keep going, but I think you get the idea.

My child was never a child in a sense. He struggled with friendships spending most of his time alone. He felt more comfortable around adult intelligence. Other kids did not seem to be intellectually on the same page as he was.

We were scared as parents of our own child. He would have tantrums that could be heard down the street from our home.

He was seven when he put a knife to his throat. He would also sneak out the window of our story and a half home to climb onto the roof.

He was diagnosed with ADHD and an unspecified mood disorder. It was not until just recently at the approximate age of fourteen Autism, Anxiety and Bipolar Disorder were added to his list of mental illnesses.

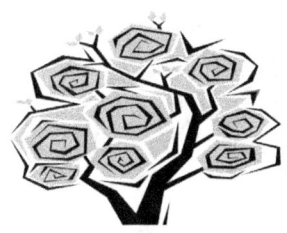

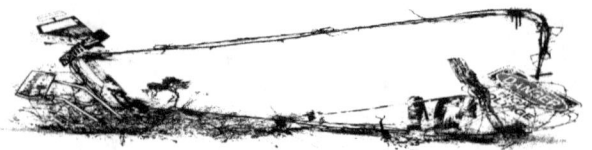

The suicide gestures still arise occasionally. I fear for my son's mental health every day. What he goes through is unimaginable, and as his mother, I feel like I have failed him in every way.

"I am unwell, and so are you.
'Help us find a way to cope.'

Struggling through each new day.
There has to be a better way.

Even with the constant cloud
Hanging over your messed-up head,
You are unique.

Raining pain
You yell so loud.

I cannot lose
The life I gave."

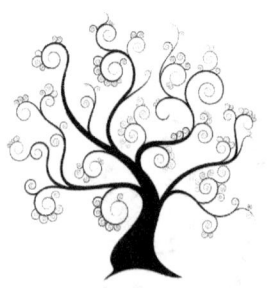

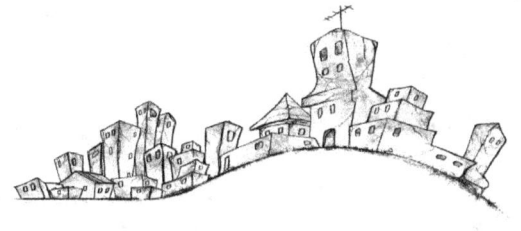

THIS IS NOT THE END

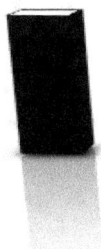

try to cope while living in a dangerous mind. In fact, learning coping mechanisms is what helps me to survive. I feel the overwhelming sensation of impending doom from anxiety.

I cannot sleep because I cannot stop thinking. It could be something someone said or something I have been procrastinating.

My heart beats out of my chest, and I cannot breathe. I am cold, and then I am hot. Everything in my body tenses up, and I become nauseous and dizzy.

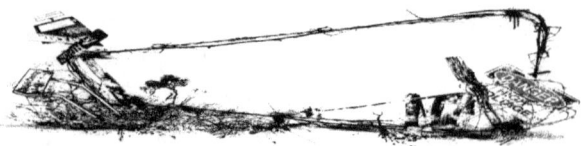

I believe the reaper will take my soul. Leading me closer to a possible alternate place, my new home.

I realize after the anxiety subsides; this is not the end. Instead, it is a piece of me that clearly does not understand how to cope with life's demands.

I started to realize that I needed goals. Things to keep my mind occupied. Long-term and short-term goals were ideal, as I lacked patience.

For a long-term goal, I would book a trip where there was sunshine to warm my face. I needed the warmth because it made me feel good inside. I am not a resort kind of girl, however. I enjoy taking snapshots of everything and learning about the culture of where I am.

Throughout elementary school and high school, I struggled in the English language and communication. I was placed in a special needs classroom in middle school because of this. I thought I was stupid because the kids told me

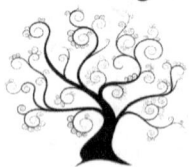

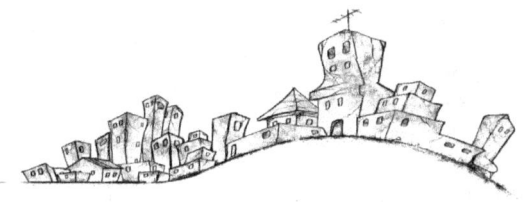

precisely that. I did manage to get the achievement award and highest mark overall in the class. Maybe I was not as intellectually challenged as I thought.

I did not believe that I could or ever would do something as intricate as writing a book. This has been years in the making because I lacked the confidence. I barely passed English class. I guess I did not think something like this could be possible. This is my very long-term goal.

My short-term goals would be as simple as saving up enough money to buy myself a pair of shoes or a new outfit. It could be a concert or a small household project.

Completing projects is a daunting task because my mind is so scattered all the time. It is essential to take medication just to finish sweeping the floor. Yes, something so simple for many is hard for me to complete.

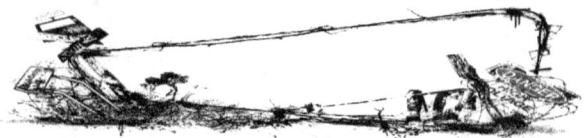

I enjoy the pictures I take because I get to edit them to the way I see the world. Unfortunately, I am a perfectionist, and nothing I do is ever good enough. I think I like a photo one day then the next I despise it. I am not sure why that is.

Every day I am different and see things in a new perspective. It could be a good thing, or it could be a bad thing. I get nothing done except spend countless hours in front of my computer, trying to make up my mind what is perfect.

I should just accept that I will never be perfect, no one is.

My sticker book was my pride and joy. It had unique stickers that I had arranged in a perfect order.

"It is gone!"

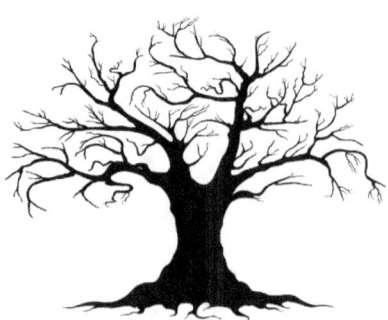

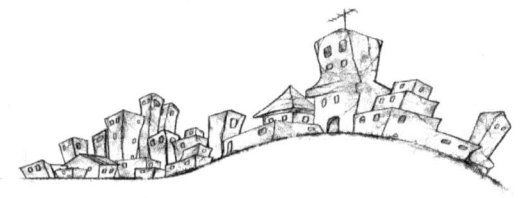

I lost the sticker book in the schoolyard one day and could not find it. It was not until the girl that sat behind me pulled it out that I realized where it went.

Finders keepers was a thing when I was young. She refused to give it back even after I begged and cried for it.

No one liked this girl, she was an outcast as well, but with a foul odour. I guess I do not blame her for not wanting to give it back. She was made fun of all through school and did not have a single friend. She was a mean girl; I am assuming as a result of all the mockery that she endured.

That sticker book was perfect, and it was gone. If I had it today, I question if I would still think it was perfect. That could have been the pivotal moment in my life that changed the way I viewed objects and everything I did and do today.

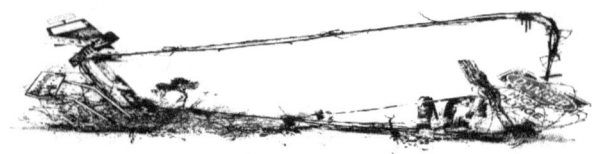

It is silly to think something so trivial could cause a life-altering domino effect, but perhaps it did.

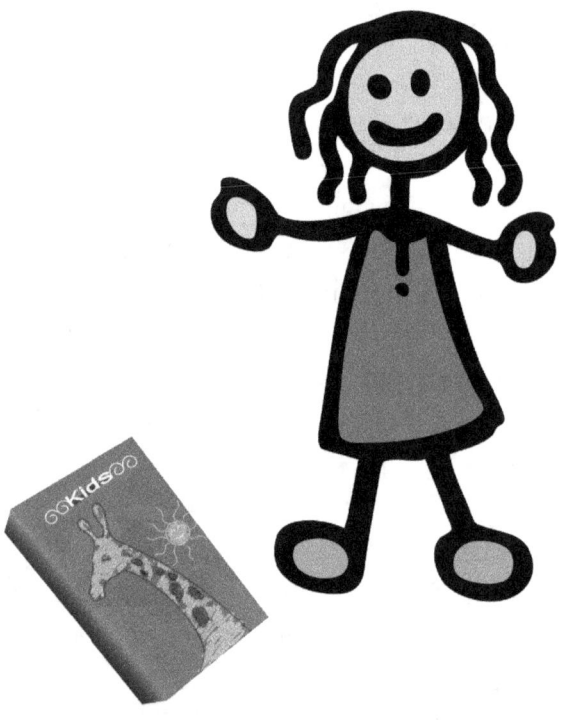

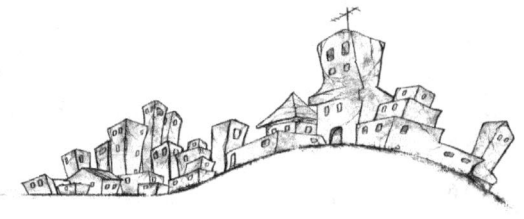

Back to the Beginning

y life began almost twenty years ago. Before that, I believed that death was a better option. I unquestionably did not think that I would be where I am today. It is far from perfect, but whose life is?

"I am washing my hair."

"I will call you back."

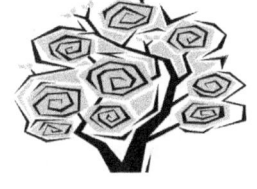

That was one of our first telephone conversations. I never called the man I met on the computer again. I completely forgot about him after the promise I made to return a simple phone call. He was going to be a big part of my life.

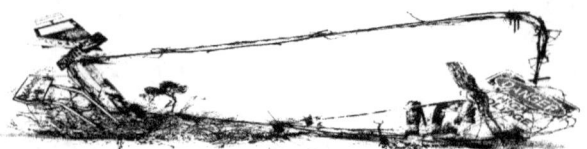

I grew up with one robust notion that the man I would spend the rest of my life with did not live in my hometown. Turns out, it was one of the only things I was right about.

I never fantasized about being a bride with a big wedding. I hate being the center of attention. A drive through marriage would be more like my dream. I like cheap and straightforward. At least that is what I keep telling myself.

I agreed to meet him for the first time on valentine's day. Long story short, he moved in the next day, and he is still the love of my life.

I remember the first time I saw him. He had dark curly hair with dark droopy eyes. His black turtle-necked sweater only amplified his eyes when they locked onto mine. The butterflies almost caused my body to collapse. I was in love, and it took less than ten seconds.

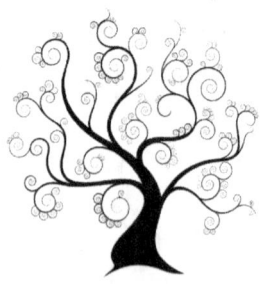

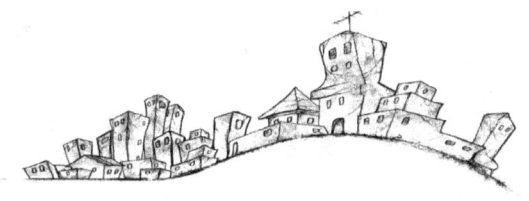

This memory is what grounds me. Love has its ups and downs and can be hard. When it gets tough, this is what I remember. The butterflies that once occupied my insides return and puts my love back into perspective. It starts with that first powerful thought, then additional memories return, further solidifying where my life truly began.

He saved me and kept me breathing all these years. His strength picked me back up every time I fell.

My wrists bleed from time to time, but the blood never runs dry when he is around.

I do not always think that I am lucky or strong. I am compelled to believe that my life is worthless. Even with love, I have often taken it for granted. I often sabotage the relationship by being cold and distant. I am afraid that I will get hurt; therefore, the wall keeps getting rebuilt.

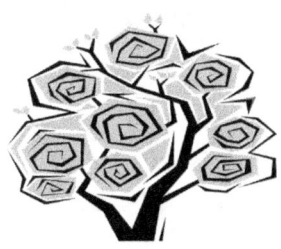

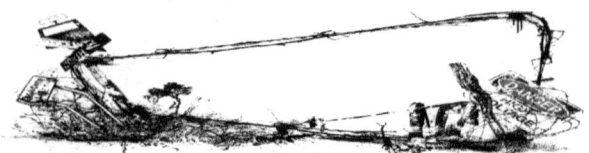

We have hurt each other countless times, but luckily, we have seen the error of our ways. The right love can make all the difference when dealing with mental illness.

Without him, I would be dead, and that is the brutal truth!

"Love can be blind.
Love can be cruel.

But love can make you strong
To help you move on.

Look past the pain,
Expose your heart.
Place it in your hand.

Believe you deserve more.
You do not need to be apart.

Share your life,
The love will set you free."

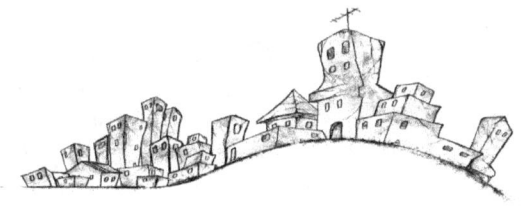

WHAT IS NEGATIVE CAN BE POSITIVE

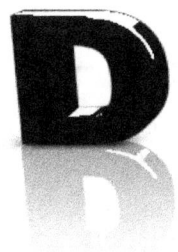

o not use mental illness as an excuse because you are better than the reason you make up. Discover what you are great at because you are imaginative, and you might not even know it.

"Fight to live because you are worth it. You will always be worth fighting for, never forget that."

"I have had many dreams.
To be a writer, I must write.
To be a photographer, I must take the photographs.

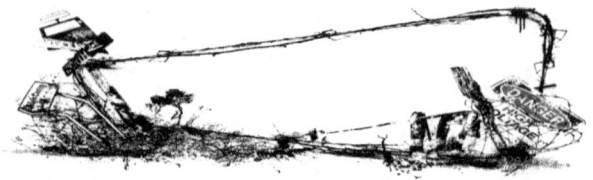

If I add the passion and dedication,
It will support my path to freedom."

Become the writer with your words to express the torment that rages inside. Show the world you are more than your mental illness. Your perspective is unique to who you are.

The journey I took you on has opened my eyes. I cannot blame others for my pain. I cannot blame mental illness because it is part of who I am. Treat it like a gift. It is all but your own.

Without mental illness, I would not see the world the way I do.

The right medications balance the predators that invade inside my head. Slowing my thoughts to a near-normal pace. Most importantly, I am still the person I was born to be.

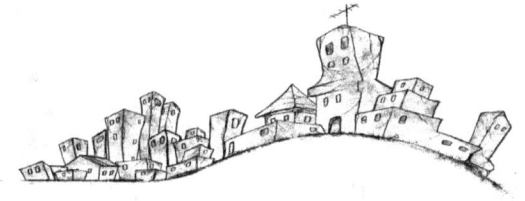

I can sit here to tell you my tale. I wanted to be a superhero with superpowers. Maybe my interpretation of a superhero was different than what is on the television or in the movies.

I realized that my dream was to help others. I will always struggle with mental illness, and so will you or someone you love. It does not go away, but that is okay. Having the right support system in place will make the difference in someone with mental illness. It is like a lifeline that holds you up when you are down. Someone to pull you from the raging fires of the unknown.

I am broken and will always be broken, but I do not want to be fixed. I do not want to be entirely fixed because it would take away who I am. I am a woman who has a mental illness, and I will always need help to survive.

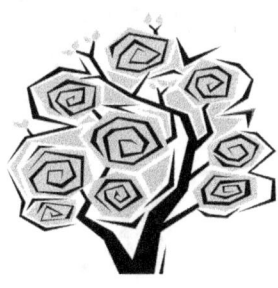

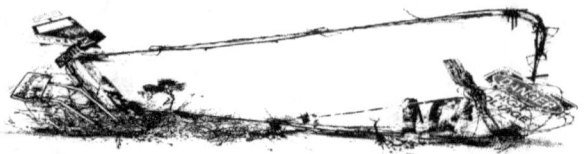

Somewhere in the middle, I began a story. I do not want to be a sheep that society controls. I do not want to be like everyone else. I want to see the portal so it can take me on adventures to see my life as I investigate the magical mirror.

Darkness may fall upon my soul. Casting a shadow where the voices cry out. I will try to escape to break free from its hold.

Rejection is part of life but remembering the blue rubber ring and the love from a stranger warms my heart.

I will walk across a rope balancing the choices that I make. I will be labelled and ridiculed because I see the pink elephants on parade.

Into the void, it swallows me whole, but I will fight in the never-ending war.

The wall that I have built towers beyond the sky, protecting from the enemy that hovers nearby.

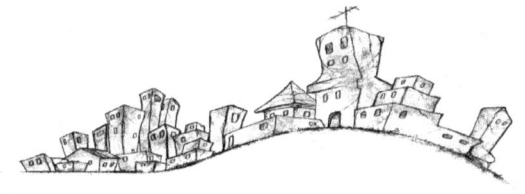

I will run away because of the darkness and the gloom.

Where are we now?

I think we have found the in-between where nothing is seen unless you believe it is real.

I see the dead people they are all around. They live in the past and walk the world today.

I am isolated within my mind. A place I created all on my own. Is it reality or illusion that my eyes project to my brain?

Where do I go from here?

This is not the end?

I will go back to the beginning and recount all the memories. What is negative can be positive.

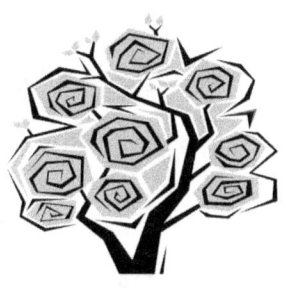

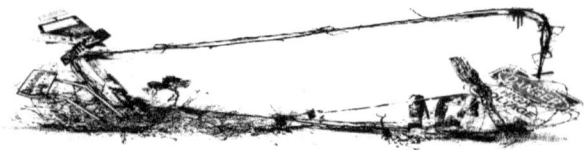

It is up to you and me to make our own dreams come true. This is not the end; instead, it is a new beginning to a life that you thought was not worth living.

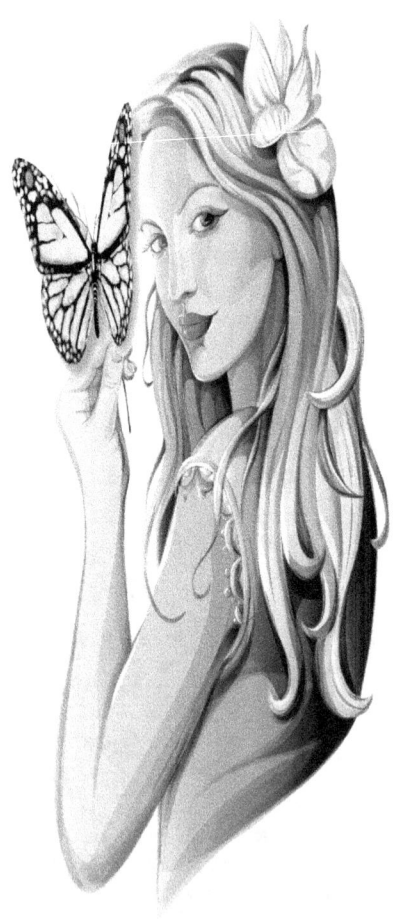

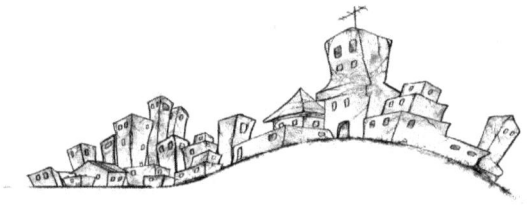

"Knowledge is the influence that stands between the battle of all that is good and evil."

- Lori S Moore

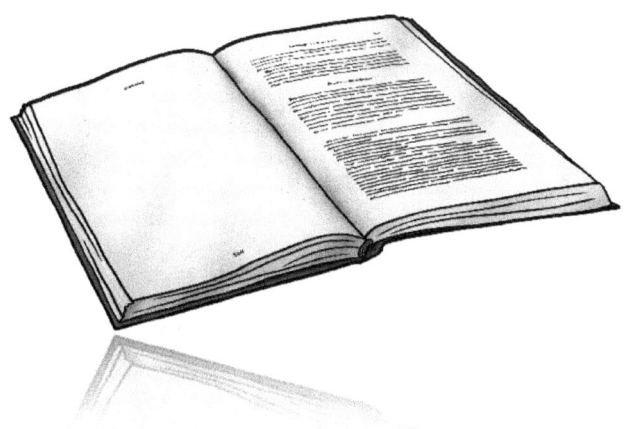